MW01029945

"This brave book helps us meet life in spite of the fact—or because of face up to mortality, grief and loss courage is our key to dying with grace, and living with passion and joy. Bless them for their gentle candor and good humor with life's greatest lessons."

Barbara Coombs Lee, President, Compassion & Choices

"Everything Leah and Nick say and share with their readers is so right on the money. The tribute to Nick's wife is wonderful, and reading both sides was inspiring. I'm sure it will help those who read it that have second guessed themselves about the decisions they made to find some peace from their story. I really couldn't put this book down."

Anne D'Ambrosio, Executive Director, Grief Recovery for all Bereaved

"Leah Vande Berg's writing reflects the thorough understanding of the situation gained from her personal experience with ovarian cancer. Her willingness to relate her perceptions to others who face the daunting prospect of her disease reflects her generous personality and thoughtfulness in the face of extraordinary adversity. Her words and hopeful spirit can guide and inspire others and their families who must cope with the same challenge."

Jonathan S. Berek, MD, MMS, Professor and Chair, Department of Obstetrics and Gynecology, Stanford University School of Medicine & Stanford Cancer Center

"Leah and Nick have written an excellent book about a very difficult journey . . . one that most of us will take. It is a very human and warm book, not an overly emotional book. There is an honesty in the description of Nick's feeling about Leah's illness and transition. The love of friends and family come through in the writing. We all have something to learn about our own journey by reading this book."

Jim Baltzell, MD, Editor Beyond Indigo

"My mother's diagnosis of ovarian cancer changed my life, and Nick's story about love, loss and going on with life after the pain was quite familiar. The family of ovarian cancer is large and passionate. Nick's story as a husband adds another dimension to our common phases of disbelief, anger, fear, sadness and yes, ultimately, finding our way through the other end. The experience of helping someone you love through the phases of dying is the most life-changing and painful experience one could ever have. Nick has allowed us to watch his process and Leah's influence in his new life. My mom and Leah are likely smiling down at us."

Deborah Ortiz, former California State Senator who sponsored legislation creating a women's gynecological cancer information program in the California Department of Health Services and establishing September as Gynecological Cancer Awareness Month.

"As I read *Cancer and Death: A Love Story in Two Voices*, I had the sense of being an invisible presence in the lives of two friends of mine while they met, fell in love, and took an incredible journey that would take one of them away from us all. It is not common to be able to 'hear' both sides of the experience, and that makes this book a rich and rewarding resource for others going though cancer. Together they have created a book that is both difficult to read and difficult to put down."

Marlene von Friederichs-Fitzwater, Ph.D., Assistant Adjunct Professor, Hematology/Oncology, UC Davis School of Medicine, and Director, Outreach Research & Education Program, UC Davis Cancer Center

"Nick and Leah's book offers incredible insight into the human side of having cancer. They tell a story of life, death, grief, and hope, not only for themselves, but for the relationship they built. It is not a story of mystical healing or a commentary on cancer care in the United States, but rather a realistic portrayal of one couple's journey as they struggled against the cancer, their own feelings, and each other, to battle the disease."

Paula R. Sherwood, RN, Ph.D., CNRN, Assistant Professor, School of Nursing, University of Pittsburgh

"Vande Berg and Trujillo offer a stirring account of their lives as they negotiate the process of cancer. Providing perspectives from multiple viewpoints, (scholars, partners, lovers, patient, care-giver), *Cancer and Death: A Love Story in Two Voices* is a genuine reflection on how cancer is an insidious interference in the lives of loved ones. The narrative that unfolds has much to offer anyone striving to get a better understanding of how cancer changes lives, how communication adapts, and how we come to realize, as one author stresses, 'not to take anything for granted.' This book is a must read for health communication students as well as those studying relational processes."

Dan O'Hair, Ph.D., Professor of Communication, University of Oklahoma

"I applaud Leah and Nick's courage to write about death and dying, a topic that gets so little attention. Their story is important as it gives voice to the experiences that are shared among families, friends, and those with cancer and terminal illness—experiences that we still know so little about. This book also provides an opportunity to engage in important dialogue about death and dying when individuals are faced with a life-threatening illness. Their experiences will likely help others manage the uncertainty of a cancer diagnosis and the shared journey of illness and death."

Elaine Wittenberg-Lyles, Ph.D., Assistant Professor of Communication Studies, University of North Texas

Cancer and Death

HEALTH COMMUNICATION
Gary L. Kreps, *series editor*

Communication in Recovery: Perspectives on Twelve-Step Groups
   Lynette S. Eastland, Sandra L. Herndon, & Jeanine R. Barr (eds.)

Communicating in the Clinic: Negotiation Frontstage and Backstage
   Teamwork
   Laura L. Ellingson

Media-Mediated Aids
   Linda K. Fuller (ed.)

Cancer-Related Information Seeking
   J. David Johnson

Changing the Culture of College Drinking: A Socially Situated
   Health Communication Campaign
   Linda C. Lederman & Lea P. Stewart

Handbook of Communication and Cancer Care
   Dan O'Hair, Gary L. Kreps, & Lisa Sparks (eds.)

Crisis Communication and the Public Health
   Matthew Seeger & Timothy Sellnow (eds.)

Cancer, Communication and Aging
   Lisa Sparks, Dan O'Hair, & Gary L. Kreps (eds.)

Cancer and Death: A Love Story in Two Voices
   Leah Vande Berg & Nick Trujillo

forthcoming

A Natural History of Family Cancer: Interactional Resources for
   Managing Illness
   Wayne Beach

Communicating Spirituality in Health Care
   Maggie Wills (ed.)

Cancer and Death

A Love Story in Two Voices

Leah Vande Berg and Nick Trujillo

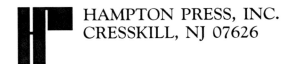
HAMPTON PRESS, INC.
CRESSKILL, NJ 07626

Printed in the United States of America

Library of Congress Cataloging-in-Publication Data

Vande Berg, Leah.
   Cancer and death : a love story in two voices / Leah Vande Berg and Nick Trujillo.
      p. cm. — (Health Communication)
   ISBN 978-1-57273-851-5 (paperbound)
   1. Vande Berg, Leah.   2. Trujillo, Nick, 1955–   3. Cancer—Patients—United States—Biography.   4. Cancer—Patients—Family relationships.   I. Trujillo, Nick, 1955–   II. Title.

RC265.6.V35A3 2008
362.196'9940092—dc22
[B]   2008026032

Hampton Press, Inc.
23 Broadway
Cresskill, NJ 07626

Contents

Acknowledgments   vii

1   A Stomach Ache in October   1

2   Beginnings   3

3   First Loves and Losses   13

4   California Loving   19

5   Life Changes   29

6   The Shock of a Lifetime   41

7   Surgery and Recovery   55

8   Chemo Reality   75

9   Back With a Vengeance   89

10 Uv Ü   107

11 Death Work   119

12 Communal Grief, Joyous Grief   135

13 Life Really Does Go On   153

Acknowledgments

When someone you love is diagnosed with a terminal illness, many people come forward to help—some quite unexpectedly—while other people you assume will be there seem to disappear. We were fortunate to have many friends and relatives help us during the most challenging period of our lives, and we wish to thank them for their support. Members of our families were always there for us, especially Leah's father Morry and her step-mother Hilly, her brother Kevin and her sister-in-law Deb, her niece Anna Leah and her nephew Austin, and her cousins Linda and Marcia as well as my mother Claudia, sister Lisa and brother-in-law Lenny, Aunt Robyn and Ed, Uncle Chuck and Aunt Penny, and my cousins Cathy, Pat and Nancy, and Tom and Kim.

Leah always considered her students to be her children, and although I do not share that view, I forever will be indebted to my "step-daughters" Jillian Tullis Owen and Juliane Mora for helping me take care of Leah while I continued to teach.

Kimo Ah Yun and Catherine Puckering offered their support for us every step of the way, as did our neighbors Dee-Dee, George, and Irene Blancet.

Laurie St. Aubin visited several times and offered to give us her airline miles so we could travel first-class to the Netherlands, if only Leah had been well enough.

Cal and Susan Galliano offered support and friendship, and they gave us their home as a sanctuary on several occasions.

Pastors Keith DeVries and Carol Pagelson provided spiritual support and friendship.

Don Kendrick organized the early Christmas Carol concert in front of our house, and he and Jim McCormick dedicated a Sacramento Choral society concert in Leah's honor.

Diego Bonilla videotaped the Christmas carol night and the funeral service, and he scanned photographs for a slide show in Leah's honor as well as for this book. Jenny Stark also videotaped the Christmas carols and helped get the poster-sized image of Leah for the funeral service.

Acknowledgments

Leah's former graduate students Sheryl Hurner, Rona Halualani, Anne Bialowas, Jay Clarkson, and Heather Hundley offered support as did our department colleagues, especially Kimo Ah Yun, Sylvia Fox, Marlene von Friederichs-Fitzwater, Diego Bonilla, Chris Miller, Josh Guilar, Virginia Kidd, Timi Poeppelman, Steve Jenkins, Bill Owen, Jenny Stark, Edith LeFebvre, Nick Burnett, Ray Koegel, Mike Fitzgerald, John Williams, Linda Tucker, Becky LaVally, Shari Lasher, Aleta Carpenter, Gerri Smith, Dave Zuckerman, Steve Buss, Lori O'Laughlin, Maggie Fuchs, Peggy Allen, and others.

Sandra Goodall created for Leah a beautiful book of photos and messages from our friends.

Bill Owen allowed us to use his haibun, titled "Horizons," from his book *Small Events*, published by Red Moon Press (redmoonpress.com).

Bob Avery took the photo of the Leah scattering at China Beach in San Francisco that appears on the back cover. Tom Trujillo took the photo of Leah in front of her "Little Red sports car and Catherine Douglas took the photo of me at Jim Morrison's grave in Paris, France. I took the front cover photo of the "Leah Cove" in Fort Bragg, California on the day I scattered her ashes there. I thank the unknown family and friends who took other photographs for the book.

Although we kept their names anonymous for medical privacy, Leah's primary care physician, surgeon, oncologist, and her surgical and oncology nurses were wonderful throughout this ordeal.

We thank the following people for sharing their voices in the book, listed in order of their appearance: Kevin Vande Berg, Lisa Holiday, Morry Vande Berg, Claudia Trujillo, Barb Rhame, Stu Heinecke, Jeff Bineham, Elsie Alcaraz, Larry Wenner, Patty Sotirin, Alex Albanese, Peggy Meyer, Pat Longan, Kimo Ah Yun, Jillian Tullis Owen, Juliane Mora, Thom McCain, Warren Press, Virginia Kidd, Mary Wall, Carol Pagelson, Mike Motley, Catherine Puckering, Peter Ehrenhaus, Janellen Hill, Laurie St. Aubin, Don Kendrick, Anna Leah Vande Berg, Bill Owen, David Zuckerman, Sylvia Fox, Diego Bonilla, Patricia Geist-Martin, Harry Haines, Greg Bowman, Susan Galliano, Chris Miller, Sheryl Hurner, Rona Halualani, Jan Andersen, Cathy Trujillo, Steve Jenkins, A. Susan Owen, Marlene von Friederichs-Fitzwater, Pat Trujillo, and Lauren Barton.

We thank Gary Kreps, the editor of the series in which this book appears, for his support, and to Barbara Bernstein and the people at Hampton Press who worked on the book.

We thank Bruce Gronbeck and the Department of Communication Studies at the University of Iowa for organizing the Leah Vande Berg Alumni Lecture in Media Studies, and we thank A. Susan Owen and Sarah Stein, co-authors of a book with Leah titled *Bad Girls: Cultural Politics and Media Representations of Transgressive Women* that was published after her death

Acknowledgments

(Peter Lang, 2007), for giving the public lectures at the very first event. We thank members of the Graduate Committee in the Department of Communication Studies at Sacramento State University and Peggy Allen and Carly Eggleston for administering the Leah Vande Berg Graduate Scholarship in Communication Studies at Sac State.

We thank everyone who contributed to these two funds in Leah's honor. Although both of these funds are endowed, tax-deductible donations are still needed and we invite readers to contribute to one of these funds.

For the IOWA fund, please make checks out to the University of Iowa Foundation, and send to the University of Iowa Foundation, P.O. Box 4550, Iowa City, IA 52244. Please note the Leah Vande Berg Lecture on the check or on a short note.

For the SAC STATE fund, please make checks out to the CSUS Trust Foundation, and send c/o the Department of Communication Studies, Sacramento State University, CA 95819. Please note the Leah Vande Berg Graduate Scholarship on the envelope and on the check or on a short note.

Finally, we thank Ebbie and Hawkeye for being wonderful companion dogs for us when we needed them the most.

1

A Stomach Ache in October

I do not recall exactly when I first felt the pain in my abdomen. I had experienced a dull ache in that region for at least a couple of weeks. I thought it was a bladder or urinary infection that would go away. My yearly physical was scheduled to take place a few weeks later, and I figured I could wait until then to tell the doctor about it. In the meantime, I continued with my busy life teaching classes, grading papers, and doing administrative work as a professor for California State University, Sacramento.

Then the pain intensified. I always have had an extremely high tolerance for pain. I think it comes from my Dutch Calvinist upbringing in small-town Iowa, where we were taught never to whine, but always to grin and bear it. I also had gained about 7 pounds that year, which I simply attributed to not exercising enough. One morning I was walking with Nick and the boys along the nearby American River Parkway on what had become our regular 5-mile route. "The boys" are our golden retriever, Ebbet, whom Nick named after Ebbets' Field, and Wheaten terrier, Hawkeye, whom I named after the mascot of my alma mater, the University of Iowa. When we crossed a bridge relatively soon after we began, I felt a searing pain in my abdomen. I doubled over and it went away, temporarily. We walked a little farther and the pain returned. I told Nick that I could not continue, and we went home. The pain subsided to a low level of discomfort when I lay down on the couch in the living room.

The next day I was very uncomfortable, but I went to school and taught my classes. Two days later, however, the pain became even more pronounced. I decided not to wait for my physical and called my personal care physician's office. The nurse recommended that I go to the hospital's lab and have some blood tests done. A doctor looked at the results and said they showed I was a little anemic, but there was no indication of any bladder or urinary infections. He said the pain could be any one of a number of things and that I should go home and call again if it persisted.

The pain became really acute during the next couple of days, and I tossed and turned every night. I called the doctor's office again and told the nurse that I was in a humongous amount of pain and needed to see someone immediately. The doctor called back several minutes later and said the pain could indicate appendicitis and that I should go to the hospital. He needed to order a bunch of tests that could take weeks if I scheduled a regular appointment, and I still would be in pain. In the emergency room, they would be able to do all of the tests and get the results immediately.

Nick was getting ready to teach his afternoon classes, and I told him that I needed to go to the hospital to get tests done. He asked if I needed a ride, but I said I could drive. I kissed him goodbye and took something to read.

Given Leah's tendency to gut out just about everything, she probably felt some soreness in her stomach for at least a few weeks before she sought medical attention. She didn't even mention it until she couldn't continue on our walk that morning.

I also had noticed that her abdomen was a bit more bloated than during the past few years, although I didn't think it unusual for a nearly 54-year-old woman. I couldn't criticize Leah for her shape because at age 47 my belly protruded more than I desired.

But when she buckled over on our walk, I knew something was wrong. Leah rarely complained about anything—she called in sick just a few times during her entire career—and I pleaded with her to go to the doctor *that day*. She countered that she could wait until her physical.

Frustrated by what I heard as her typically stubborn response, I said, "What if you have a tumor or something serious?"

She insisted that she had a bladder infection, and then we debated her qualifications to make such a diagnosis.

I was relieved when she finally went to the hospital a few days later. When I kissed her before going to Sacramento State to teach my afternoon and evening classes, I assumed she would get some tests done and receive medication for a bladder infection or intestinal problem.

I came home around 8:30 that night, but Leah was not there. She had left a message on the answering machine to call her at the hospital.

The hospital operator took several minutes to connect me to the room, but Leah finally answered.

"Mr. Nickers," she said calmly, using the nickname she coined for me several years earlier. "They think I have cancer."

2

Beginnings

Leah and I didn't spend a lot of time with each other growing up because I was involved in sports and she was always reading or doing schoolwork. But she was my big sister, so she always looked out for me. Anytime I'd get in trouble for breaking a window with a baseball she would come to my defense.

(Leah's brother, Kevin)

I grew up in Sioux Center, a small town near the northwest corner of Iowa. My little brother, Kevin, and I were among its 2,500 residents in the 1950s and 1960s.

Our community revolved around church. Back then the people in town were almost 100 percent of Dutch ancestry, and pretty much everybody was Dutch Reformed, Christian Reformed, or Reformed, all variations of Calvinist theology. I was raised Reformed, the most liberal doctrinally, but there were many strict Dutch Reformed people in town who wore Amish-looking clothes and believed that most human pleasures were evil, wicked, and sinful. As a result, Sioux Center did not have a movie theatre, we called school dances "rhythm games" because dancing was forbidden, and the only place that sold beer was Joe's Tavern.

My mom, Norma, was the school superintendent's secretary. She worked at the office at school, so I would bop in every day to say hello. If I ever forgot anything, she would leave work and walk the few blocks to our house to get it. She saved me on numerous occasions when I failed to bring my homework to school.

My dad, Morry, was a letter carrier in town, and later he delivered mail on the rural route to outlying communities. He left for work really early in the morning and had finished by the time the school day ended, so he was the one at home in the afternoons. He would watch us play baseball in the backyard, and he kept fixing the windows of the garage that we kept breaking. In the summertime, he played adult league baseball with his former high school buddies, and after games they sometimes would have a beer.

Like most people in town, my parents were very stoic. They did not hug and kiss and cry that much, and they did not create scenes. You were supposed to be able to control yourself. If you were happy, you were not supposed to gloat, and if you were sad, you were not supposed to mope.

My parents did not have much money, so we lived in rented houses early on. We finally bought our own house on Fourth Avenue, which was a big deal for us. I remember my Aunt Ruth helped my mom and I wallpaper my room with beautiful purple paper. Mom was great about letting me re-decorate my room every few years. We could not afford expensive material, but we did really creative things with what we had.

An old oil-burning stove near the dining room generated the heat for the house. In the winter, I would get up really early and sit in the bathroom in front of a vent. That was my favorite place to study because I was not disturbing anybody and it was so nice and warm.

School was very important, and one of my life gifts was that my parents truly valued education. The one thing you could get out of any chore for was studying.

I especially loved to read. Sioux Center was very safe, and I could walk to the library by myself to get books. I read way above my grade level, but the librarian would not let me check out certain books until my mother signed a card saying I could read all of them, whether they were for children or adults. By reading books, I could go anywhere in the world and I could be any one of the different characters that led all these exiting and exotic lives. I absolutely inhaled books.

Music was very important as well. I played flute and piccolo in the concert band and I was a majorette in the marching band, but I loved to sing. Singing was a form of emotional and poetic expression, especially singing hymns. They were about ideas and emotions, and some of them were quite powerful and evocative. My mom and I also sang together when we did dishes. She was really good at harmony. We would sing songs that were popular from her youth, like "Sweet Adeline" and "Down by the River." I had a little beige and red 78-rpm record player, and I sang along with the records.

I wanted to play the piano, but my parents could not afford a piano. I went and asked the deacons at church if I could practice several half hours over the course of the week in return for doing whatever they wanted me to do around there. They agreed, and I did that until my parents saved up enough money for a piano, which I got to have in my bedroom. That was the only place it could fit, but it was wonderful because that meant I could play my piano pretty much anytime I wanted to, unless everyone was sleeping. My parents were wonderfully encouraging and supportive about music.

In grade school, only boys played sports. They started girls track and softball as intramural sports when I was in high school. They did not yet have girls' basketball.

I was a very religious kid. I thought about God a lot, and I read my Bible and prayed every day. I learned all of the Bible stories: Abraham warning his brother Lot about Sodom and Gomorrah so they could leave, and Lot's wife looking back and being turned into a pillar of salt. The good shepherd puts 99 sheep in the fold and goes out looking for the lost one. These and other stories told me that when God says something you should really listen because he means it. But God also is loving and merciful. He gives you chances to escape. He goes out looking for one lost soul, wanting everyone to be safe and loved.

We prayed before every meal, whether at home or at a restaurant. My dad always made up a prayer before we ate dinner, and then he would say, "Whoever eats the fastest gets the mostest." He read from the Bible at the end of the meal.

My parents encouraged me to argue with them about religion and to take different views. They sometimes would get a little taken aback by how far I questioned things, but they never discouraged me from asking hard questions and trying to find answers to them.

I remember reading to Nicky when he was a little boy. He just gobbled up everything. He sang all the nursery rhymes. His favorite was a book called "The Bumper Book." There was one story about an elephant that he thought was hysterical.

When I was on the road with his dad in Chicago we bought him a little jukebox from my Aunt. He loved that jukebox. He would dance and sing. He was very animated. He loved the song "Bah Bah Black Sheep," but because he was so little and hadn't developed his language skills yet he sounded Chinese when he would sing it. It was very funny.

(Nick's mom, Claudia)

I once told Leah that we had the same small-town upbringing, although I grew up in Las Vegas, Nevada. My parents moved there from Los Angeles in 1960 when I was 4 years old and my sister Michelle was 2; my youngest sister, Lisa, was born a year later. My father Bill, a tenor sax player with Stan Kenton's big band at the time, wanted to stay home with his kids and wife Claudia, a devout Catholic of Polish descent. My dad played in the orchestra at the Tropicana, the Stardust, and other hotels, and my mom worked from time to time as a secretary to bring in extra money.

Even with gambling and showgirls on "The Strip," Vegas felt like a small town in the 1960s and 1970s, and it was a great place to raise a family with good wages, cheap houses, and clean air. I attended Our Lady of Las Vegas Elementary School—honestly—and grew up Catholic in "Sin City." I'm still trying to untangle the consequences of that contradiction.

My family lived in an apartment near the Sahara Hotel and then in a rented house near downtown before we bought our own house by Twin Lakes in the northwest part of town. A few years later, the city evicted our entire block to make room for a freeway, and my parents bought a home with a similar floor plan two houses away on Eldorado Street. I'll always remember when my mom woke up Mishe, Lisa, and me to watch a big rig haul away our Austin Avenue house.

Unlike Leah's family, the Trujillo household rarely was stoic. We hugged and kissed and cried and yelled. Family scenes were regular occurrences. On more than one occasion, I engineered a way to get grounded in the peaceful sanctuary of my room to escape the drama.

My early childhood also revolved around church, school, and music, although I played sports as well. By the time I started Our Lady, the Dominican nuns, who wore their heavy penguin suits even in the desert heat, didn't smack kids on the knuckles with rulers anymore. They made up for the lack of physical discipline with guilt, mortification, and images of burning in hell for eternity or Purgatory for millennia.

I served as an altar boy from grades 6 to 8. In the sixth and seventh grades, I devoted myself to God and vowed to become a priest, although they had to remain celibate. Then I developed a crush on Sandy LaPointe in eighth grade, and my plans changed. By the end of eighth grade, my fellow altar boy veterans and I were drinking sacramental wine and selling unblessed hosts to second graders for 10 cents a pop, three for a quarter.

My family prayed before every meal, although we speed-recited the standard "Bless-us-oh-Lord-and-these-thy-gifts-which-we-are-about-to-receive-from-thy-bounty-through-Christ-our-Lord-Amen" without taking a breath. Every year a priest blessed our Easter basket, which always housed my mom's Lamb of God butter sculpture, except for the year I dropped the lam o'butter on its head in the parking lot. We went to church every Sunday and on every Holy Day of Obligation, including January First for the Circumcision of Christ, although my parents never explained what that meant. The reason didn't matter—if it was a Holy Day of Obligation, you went to mass.

My parents and teachers discouraged us from questioning any Catholic beliefs. I remember when Sister Seamus Ann, my eighth-grade teacher at Our Lady, sent me to the principal's office when I challenged the idea that God wouldn't allow unbaptized babies in heaven. I thought it was totally unfair that they had to spend eternity in Limbo because they didn't have their original sin washed away. When I refused to attend church in my teens, my parents grounded me to my room.

In a household led by a jazz musician, music was vital. Like other kids my age, I listened to the Beatles, the Rolling Stones, and Jimi Hendrix, but I also enjoyed Charlie Parker, Stan Getz, and other jazz greats on my dad's LPs.

Jazz talk filled our home and our lives. My dad and his musician friends called each other "cats" and their wives "chicks." If my dad didn't like someone, he was a "jive turkey." Something good was "groovy," whereas something bad was a "drag" or "strictly B-flat." He used "man" to punctuate almost every sentence, as in "Don't be a drag, man."

My sisters and I sang in our grade-school choirs and took piano lessons from Mrs. Purney, a quaint authoritarian who seemed to be 100 years old. At age 13, I took guitar lessons for a year. I didn't stick with that either, although I've taken up guitar again in my 50s.

School was very important in our family. My mom read to us when we were very young, and she insisted that we go to Catholic elementary and high school to get a good education. I am convinced that my mom is responsible for my early interest and ongoing success in school.

My dad played catch with me and made sure I owned the best equipment. I participated in organized baseball, basketball, and soccer in grade school and virtually every sport on the street with George, David, Butchie, and my next-door neighbor and best friend, Jay.

At age 10, I saw a science fiction matinee with Jay and George, two friends on the block. Later that night, the three of us played "mad scientists" by filling with gasoline a plastic bottle that Jay's Aunt Clara used for hair dye. We lit the tip and squeezed, launching flames into the vacant lot next to Jay's home where my family's house used to be.

The last time we lit the top, the entire bottle exploded, knocking George and me to the ground. When we sat up, we saw Jay, on fire from his waist up, running around the lot screaming.

George and I threw dirt on Jay to put out the flames to no avail. After a horrifying minute or two, he finally fell, and we patted down his smoldering chest with our tee shirts because he was too hot to touch with our hands. Jay's dad was working his shift as a fireman at the Nevada Test Site 60 miles away, so George's dad drove Jay to the hospital. Over 50% of Jay's body was badly burned, and he was given "extreme unction"—the last rites—multiple times. Somehow he survived and recovered, and we remained friends until we drifted apart in high school. I always thought that incident in October 1966 would be the worst experience I ever went through in my life. It was until Leah got cancer in the same month, 37 years later.

In high school, Leah was very active in a lot of things. She sang in choirs, and she read a lot with a neighbor lady. She also had a lot of boyfriends. Some of them almost broke her heart.

(Leah's dad, Morry)

I was a little Miss Goody-Two-Shoes in high school. I did not drink or smoke cigarettes, and drugs were unheard of back then. The calendar might have read the 1960s, but it felt like 1950 in Sioux Center. The only trouble I faced was for having my skirt too short and my bangs not cut two inches above my eyebrows. The closest I came to sex was kissing or petting with my boyfriends.

I was the salutatorian of my class. Another girl was the valedictorian because she only took home economics classes, whereas I took calculus and trigonometry. I thought it singularly unfair that the As in her easy classes counted the same as the As in my difficult classes. They let me give a speech at graduation anyway, and my parents were very proud.

I wanted to be a missionary doctor because my mom's aunt was a missionary in India. I was moved emotionally by her letters, and I really felt that I had been called to minister to poor and sick people in India. I did really well in my chemistry and biology classes, but I took an anatomy class in which we had to experiment on animal cadavers. I do not know whether medicine was what I was supposed to have done with my life, but cutting up God's creatures clearly was not something I could do. I moved to my second choice, which was to be an English teacher, because I loved literature.

My parents had to approve all of the boys I dated. I always liked older boys. During my freshman year, I went out with Wayne Evanhois and David Haarscamp. Then I started dating Kenneth Vande Berg, no relation, the summer after my freshman year. He was going to become a minister, and my parents thought that was swell. His career plans did not preclude us from kissing hot and heavily. I waffled back and forth with Ken for some time, but he was getting ready to leave for college so that relationship ended.

During my junior year, I met Barry Ekdom at the Sioux County music festival. He was 2 years older than me and was a handsome rakish lad. I thought he was hot stuff, and I really fell for him. We talked on the phone a couple of times, and I went out with him. My mom and dad, however, were not wild about him. He was from Orange City, our rival town 10 miles away, so they did not know everything about him. Then one of my teachers reported to my parents that Barry and his friends were caught drinking beer at the state basketball tournament, and my dad told me that I could not see him anymore. They thought they were doing the right thing, but I was convinced that Barry was being maligned by this gossipy self-righteous teacher.

Although my parents did not want me to date Barry, I still sneaked telephone calls to him and visits to Orange City to see him. I remember going there one day with my friend in her father's car. When we came back to Sioux Center, we drove the car backward because we heard you could take miles off the odometer by driving backward. The town police officer stopped us and said that driving backward does not take miles off. He told me to go home and tell my parents what I had done or he would do so when my dad gassed up his car at the Phillips 66 station the next morning before his mail route. Needless to say, I was placed on restriction for a goodly time and was not allowed to go to a sock hop.

I became really angry with my parents, and we had marathon fights about Barry. They told me that they were looking out for my welfare and they wanted me to finish high school, go to college, and not throw my life away doing stupid things. My view was that I was going to college, and dating this boy was not going to change that. We went round and round like that for a while.

This battle went on throughout the summer between my junior and senior year. In the fall of my senior year, my parents finally relented. They realized that it did not matter if I dated Barry because nothing was going to get in the way of my going to college. I think they also realized that I would be on my own pretty soon and then I would do what I wanted anyway. They said I could go to the senior prom with Barry, but I could not go to the same college. Barry went to Iowa, so I would have to go to Iowa State.

———————————

I remember my brother being a kind big brother who—I'll be honest—showed a little favoritism toward me—his baby sister! Although we weren't close siblings because there was a 6-year age difference, I always looked up to Nick and was very proud of him for his good grades and his sports accomplishments. I remember Nick being calm and laid-back and only getting upset when he and my dad were at odds with one another—usually at the dinner table.

I was particularly excited when he moved out of the house because I was the recipient of his bedroom and no longer had to share a room with my big sister.

(Nick's sister, Lisa)

———————————

I was a pretty typical teenage boy in high school. During my 4 years at Bishop Gorman, I studied enough to get Bs, but I mostly played sports, especially baseball, at which I excelled as a pitcher with a wicked curveball. Leah's calling might have been to help the poor and sick in India, but mine was to pitch for the Los Angeles Dodgers.

Another passion in high school was to drink and get high with my buddies. While Leah inhaled books in Sioux Center, I inhaled marijuana in Las Vegas. I smoked my first joint at Lake Mead in the summer of 1969 before my freshman year, and over the next 4 years progressed through hash, reds, speed, mescaline, mushrooms, and LSD, although I never snorted cocaine or shot heroin, which we considered to be the most dangerous items on the drug pyramid. Sometimes we got stoned and gambled at casinos like the Thunderbird and Hacienda that allowed teens with fake IDs, but mostly we watched people gamble, especially Midwestern grandmothers in knee socks who could play 10 slots at a time. I stopped taking acid after I shattered my big toe in a soccer game when I tried to kick the ball and missed and an opponent made direct contact with my foot rather than the ball.

My parents and I never fought about my girlfriends because I did not have any steady girlfriends in high school. I was shy, had zits, and suffered extreme embarrassment whenever I picked up girls in the Rambler station wagon or Buick Skylark I inherited from my dad, both of which sputtered and shook after turning off the ignition. I did have sex in high school, although my first two experiences occurred at a legal brothel outside of the county limits near the interstate leading to St. George, Utah. My other sexual experiences were not significantly more romantic, occurring in parks and in the backseat of cars.

Although I didn't fight with my parents about dating, I experienced the typical conflicts that occur between a father and a rebellious teenager. My dad has threatened to write a book entitled *Take Out the Trash*, a reference to the battles we reenacted almost daily whenever he ordered me to take out the trash and I didn't immediately comply. He also could write *Clean Your Room, Give Me the Salt, Turn the Channel*, and other sequels in the series. I spent a lot of time on restriction in my teens.

Ironically, I learned to be defiant to authority from my dad. He said he hated his brief military stint in the 1950s because officers ordered him around. In the 1970s, he was fired by Wayne Newton when the Vegas entertainer demanded that my dad laugh at his jokes between songs and he responded, "The only thing funny about you is your [expletive deleted] singing." He drove a cab for a year after that incident.

I planned to attend the University of Wyoming, where I received a baseball scholarship. However, I found alternative funding at the University of Southern California, and I went there to pursue my dream of playing professional baseball.

3

First Loves and Losses

I loved living with Leah. We both had radical changes in our lives at the same time. I'm sure that she spent as much time helping me to adjust as I did helping her. I think she was pretty controlled about the breakup of her marriage. As a sort of humorous way of dealing with it, I remember we would plot imaginary punishments that would befall our ex-husbands. However, throughout, she remained very kind, intensely fair about settlements, and I think loving in a much broader sense than her ex could have understood. She was the most supportive and accepting person I have ever known.

(Leah's friend, Barb)

My parents drove me to Iowa State University in the fall of 1969. Although I could not wait to get there, I became desperately homesick. At the end of the first semester, I caught a severe cold, which turned into pneumonia and then mononucleosis. By January, I was so sick that I had to drop out of school. After I recovered, I told my parents I would not return to Iowa State and had decided to go to Iowa. I was a far more fragile person than I thought I was, and I needed Barry for support. My parents were not happy about my decision, but they did not want me to drop out of college, so they allowed me to attend Iowa.

My sophomore year was 1970, when campuses across the country were in an uproar protesting the Vietnam War. It was an extraordinary time. I wore mini-skirts and an army fatigue jacket and marched down Main Street with protestors. In the spring, the demonstrations kept growing, and teachers canceled classes and had sit-ins. The civil right's movement and the first "Take Back the Night" women's march also took place. Then students were killed at Kent State in May, and the president of the University of Iowa closed the campus for the rest of the year.

Barry and I definitely were in love. I had sex for the first time with him at Iowa, and it was wonderful. We decided to get engaged, and that Christmas Barry asked my dad for permission to marry me. My dad said no. When Barry told me that my dad did not approve our engagement, he had tears in his eyes. I assured my parents that I would stay in college, and I told them that I was going to marry Barry regardless of whether they supported it. They relented, and Barry and I got married the following August.

At the rehearsal dinner the night before the wedding, my mom said, "You know it's not too late to change your mind."

I told her firmly that I would not be changing my mind.

Our wedding took place in Central Reformed Church. It was a typical Sioux Center affair. The wedding occurred upstairs, and then everybody went downstairs for cake and ice cream. Then we changed our clothes and went on our honeymoon.

For the first few years, Barry and I had a great time. We were going to school and working, but we enjoyed going out, listening to live music, and playing pinnacle and 500 with our friends. He gave me an Old English Sheepdog for my graduation, whom I named Sebastian, and he proceeded to eat the stuffing out of the cushions of our brand-new sofa. He was quite a problem child, but he was my buddy.

I started my master's degree in English, also at Iowa, and worked at the library as a clerk. When I completed my M.A., I was a finalist for several teaching positions, including one that a male friend of ours received because they said he was a man with a wife and a child to support, even though I had more English hours and was better qualified for the job. That experience upset me enormously because it was singularly unfair. It is not unlikely that it marked the beginning of my feminist proclivities.

The next year, North Lynn Consolidated School, a little high school in the middle of a cornfield made up of different communities, hired me to teach English and mass media and to supervise the newspaper, the radio broadcast, and the yearbook. We moved to Cedar Rapids, and Barry found a job as a pretrial release officer. His position required more than 40 hours per week, and I taught all day and then had to work on the yearbook and newspaper at night.

Barry and I were working at different places at different times, getting home late, and not spending enough time on our relationship. I learned that you have to work to keep intimacy up, both emotional and physical intimacy. We had not been doing that because we were so focused on our work. Many nights I did not come home until 9:30 pm, and then I would have to leave the next day at 6:30 in the morning. We did not spend enough time with each other and we started to grow apart. We were not fighting or arguing; we were just distant from each other.

After teaching high school for a couple years, I decided to return to Iowa and get my Ph.D. in Communication, so we moved back to Iowa City. We still worked long hours and spent little time together, and we did not even talk to each other that much.

Barry was a graduate assistant in psychology, and he met a young woman who was an undergraduate assistant. He started having coffee with her and seeing her, and he ultimately fell in love with her. I became very angry and jealous. I followed him on my bicycle once when he drove off in our car, and I saw him meet her at a restaurant. I confronted him about it later that day and went bonkers. I thought if he saw me with someone else he would become jealous, but when I tested that theory it only made him more distant. We hung on together for almost a year, and then 2 weeks before my comprehensive exams he said he was moving out and getting his own place.

I was devastated. I knew it was coming, but I thought we would find a way to make it work. We were both young and very stubborn.

My parents were extremely distressed when Barry and I divorced. They were embarrassed because divorce was a stigma in my hometown at that time. But that was of far less concern than how absolutely sad and broken up I was. My dad bought me my first-ever new car, a snake-vomit green Volkswagen Rabbit.

I threw myself into finishing my doctorate. I found a roommate, Barb, and my Ph.D. buddies, Candy and Steve, became my support system. I took up tae kwon do and joined the university sailing club and did all kinds of activities to keep myself busy so I would be tired at night. Even with Barb in the house, it was kind of empty and I was very lonely. I took Sebastian on walks and to the park, and he cuddled with me in bed.

The following May, Candy and Steve moved to West Lafayette to work at Purdue University. I visited them on a number of weekends and met some of their graduate students and colleagues. I casually dated a professor and a graduate student at Purdue at the same time, the first time I had ever done that. Although they were pleasant diversions at first, the situation turned into a colossal disaster when the professor told the graduate student that he no longer could see me. That infuriated me, and I stopped seeing both of them.

A few weeks later, I met John, a bicycle racer and a handyman. He did some work on the apartment I was renting in Iowa City. He also was divorced, and he called and asked me out on a date. I liked him a lot. He was very different, the first nonacademic I had been involved with in a long time. I dated him for a year and a half. He even came home with me to Sioux Center once for Thanksgiving to meet my parents.

I finished my dissertation in 1981 and was hired as a professor in the Radio, Television, and Film Department at Northwestern University in Evanston, Illinois, just north of Chicago. I shared an apartment with a friend's younger sister who was about to start law school there. John came to Chicago to visit, and I would return to Iowa City to visit him. We became fairly serious and dated my whole first year at Northwestern. However, he made it unambiguously clear that he could not live in a city like Chicago, and I was not going to give up what I had spent all those years working on or trust that a relationship with a man would work out. We agreed to go our separate ways, but then we would get lonely and I would return to Iowa City to see him or he would come to Chicago to see me. We did not really want to break up, but we knew that we had to because what we wanted to be and where we wanted to be ultimately were not compatible. After dating for more than a year, we finally broke up for good, and I was alone again.

The thing I remember about Nick and Sally was how well they fit together. When you're that young, often relationships don't reach much past the obvious sexual excitement of being paired up. But Nick and Sally seemed to have a deep level of care and respect. They loved each other, but they also liked each other deeply. They were lovers and friends, all rolled into one.

(Nick's undergraduate friend, Stu)

I entered USC in the fall of 1973. I loved attending such a big-time college, where I met new friends, took challenging classes, and went to football games at the Coliseum and the Rose Bowl. I also loved living in Los Angeles, where I could visit my grandmother in East L.A. and hang out with my cousins at Manhattan Beach.

As my first semester progressed—and as my acne cleared up—I gained new self-confidence and had a couple girlfriends. Toward the end of my freshman year, I met Sally O'Donnell, a tall, athletic brunette who rowed for the USC women's crew. For our first date, we ran stairs at the Coliseum. My legs were in great shape because, contrary to common wisdom, the power in pitching is generated from the legs rather than the arm. But I learned that rowers may have the fittest legs of all athletes. I managed to keep up with Sally as she sprinted up and down those stairs, but I could barely walk the next day.

Sally and I continued to date our sophomore year and quickly became college sweethearts. We did *everything* together, including major in the same field—sociology—although I took enough courses in communication to earn a second major.

While my relationship with Sally flourished, my baseball career fizzled. I learned there is a big difference between being a scholarship player and a "walk-on." As the latter, I made the varsity squad, but pitched very little. I enjoyed a few personal highlights, including pitching against major leaguers like Fred Lynn and Steve Kemp in an alumni game, learning a knuckleball from then-Dodger pitcher Charlie Hough at Dodger Stadium, and pitching in legendary coach Rod Dedeaux's 1,001st victory. But I became bitter over my lack of playing time, and I quit the team in April of my senior year.

I was wrong to quit, but I was frustrated, embarrassed, and just plain pissed off at the world. After 15 years of defining my identity through baseball, I felt that baseball itself—through the USC coach—had betrayed me. I refused to consider the thought of being a baseball player, a baseball coach, or a baseball anything.

I remember walking to class the day after I quit the team. I had just given up on my dream and had no idea what I was going to do with my life.

Just then one of my favorite professors drove by. He was a charismatic teacher who loved the academic life. Because of him, I enjoyed going to class, doing research, and writing papers. But at that moment, he was driving his convertible sports car and wearing a tee shirt and tennis shorts on his way to play a few rounds with the beautiful coed in the passenger seat. He beamed a smile as he passed.

I waved back and decided to become a college professor.

In the final semester of our senior year, I asked Sally to marry me, and she said yes. We were married in December 1977 after the first semester of our master's programs at San Diego State University, 2 weeks after my 22nd birthday. Because we did everything together, we even hyphenated our last names to become Nick and Sally O'Donnell-Trujillo, O-T for short.

Like Leah and Barry, Sally and I focused on our work. We earned our master's degrees (Sally's in social work and mine in communication) and immediately started work on our doctorates at the University of Utah (Sally's in sociology and mine in communication).

After 3 years at Utah, Sally and I took professor positions at Purdue University. The first year in West Lafayette, Indiana, was very stressful. We mostly worked on our dissertations and adjusted to life in a small and bitter-cold Midwestern town. We started to fight with each other, but we did not take the time to work out our conflicts because we had to finish our dissertations. By the time we defended our dissertations in February 1983, there wasn't much left of our relationship. We split up that spring and divorced for "irreconcilable differences" that summer. I took back my "maiden" name and was on my own again.

4

California Loving

Nick and Leah met at a baby shower in celebration of our son's birth. Of course we didn't think anything about it at the time, since we had no idea that Nick and Leah would eventually be married. But there is a kind of irony in the situation: that at a party to celebrate the arrival of a new life, they would also begin a journey that would be their new life together.

(Friend and former graduate student, Jeff)

In the spring of 1983, I visited Candy and Steve at Purdue, and they took me to a baby shower for a graduate student and his wife. I met a new faculty member in their department named Nick and his wife, Sally. He was really cute, and I thought it too bad that he was married. I talked to his wife about the Midwest and the pressure people put on you to have kids, the difficulties of a new job in a new place, and juggling relationships and careers.

I do not remember the particulars of my conversation with Nick. I told him about my dog, and I think we talked about music. I do remember him saying that there was not much to do in Lafayette, and I told him about how much there was to do in Chicago.

That summer, Candy and Steve were coming from Purdue to Chicago to see me. They called and told me that the professor I met at the baby shower was divorced. They said they thought Nick and I would get along really well and that it might be fun for them to bring him along and we all could go to a Cubs' game together.

I told them that was a bad idea. Those little match-making endeavors never work out, and if it did not work out it would be exceedingly awkward because Nick was their colleague. So I vetoed the idea.

That November I attended the National Communication Association convention in Washington DC. For the first time, I ate soft-shelled crabs, which I thought were singularly exquisite. I attended meetings during the day and parties at night. I was walking down the hotel hallway going to a party as several people were coming out of the party. One of those people was Nick. He remembered me, and I remembered him. He said that he would be in Chicago in a couple weeks for Thanksgiving to visit his grandmother and wanted to know whether I would be willing to take him to my favorite jazz and blues clubs.

I told him I would be there and that he could give me a call, and I went into the party thinking that would be nice. However, I assumed he had drunk enough alcohol that he might not even remember talking to me. It was a convention, after all, where people drink a lot and say things they sometimes do not remember the next day.

I went home and a week or so later I received a phone call from Nick. I thought, he really is coming to Chicago for Thanksgiving and he really does want to go out with me. I thought, this is actually a man who remembers things and who follows through on what he says he is going to do.

We agreed to go out on the Friday after Thanksgiving. He came to my townhouse that night and met Rory Pooh, my Airedale. I drove my new red Rabbit and we went to Chicago to my favorite jazz, blues, and reggae clubs. We were drinking and dancing, but also talking a lot. After we closed down one club at 4:00 a.m., I was not ready for the evening to end. I asked Nick if he would like to come back to my place and continue the conversation.

It was an extraordinary first date. Nick left around 9:00 in the morning. Sleeping with somebody on the first date was not something I did, but there was some kind of magical chemistry with him. I liked him and wanted to spend more time together. He said he would call and I said great, and that is how we left it. I slept away a large part of the day to recuperate. Then I thought it might have been a mistake to sleep with him because he might never call again.

Nick did not call for several days, and I started to wonder whether he was ever going to call. Maybe five or six nights later, the phone rang and it was Nick. He told me how much fun he had and that he wanted to come to Chicago again in a few weeks to spend his birthday with me. I thought that sounded like a great idea.

I cooked Coquille St. Jacques for him, and we went out and listened to music. We came back to my place, and Nick stayed the night again. It was another wonderful date, and I knew that I really liked this guy and hoped he would keep calling.

At one point, I asked him what birthday it was for him, and he said it was his 28th. I was shocked. I was 34 at the time and was astonished that I was taken with a man who was 6 years younger than me. However, he was a professor at the same level that I was, and he also had been married before. I thought I would keep an open mind and see what unfolded.

A few weeks later, I went to Lafayette. I saw Candy and Steve, but I stayed with Nick. Then Nick came back to Chicago, and we started to date regularly.

In April, I met a female graduate student from Purdue who was teaching part time at Northwestern in the Communication Department. One day we had lunch together and she asked whether I knew Nick. I said I did, and she proceeded to tell me that he was coming to see her that weekend. That knocked the breath out of me because I realized he was dating this graduate student and me at the same time. I went home upset, not knowing what to do. I did not believe in polyamorous relationships. The previous year, I had dated two men at the same time, and it turned out to be a colossal disaster. The situation with Nick and this graduate student looked like it was shaping up to be another colossal disaster.

I called Nick and told him about my lunch with her. I said I knew that we did not have an exclusive understanding, but I was not particularly comfortable with him dating multiple women from my university where I could run into them and feel really awful. I realized I was saying that Nick could not do exactly what I had done a year earlier. It was an incredible double standard and very hypocritical. I was on the other side of the fence, and it felt rotten. I told him that if he wanted to date her that was fine, but then we would have to back off.

Nick was very calm. He said that we did not have an exclusive relationship and that dating her did not have anything to do with dating me. He said he could be dating other women at Purdue. I said I knew that, but I would not run into them there. We ended the conversation with me saying that is how I felt and with him saying he would think about what I said and get back to me.

I was not at all sure what Nick would do. He finally called me about a week later.

Now I know why you haven't written, and I'm heart-broken. What could have happened to break you and Sally apart. You had so-------- much going for you. . . .

(from Nick's grandmother's journal)

Sally and I were not doing well in the spring of 1983, but we put on a happy face to attend the baby shower for Jeff and his wife. Steve and Candy brought their friend, Leah, whom I thought was moderately attractive.

Throughout the party, Leah seemed to flirt with me, smiling widely and flashing her sparkling blue eyes. Almost any man will start or continue a conversation with a woman who flirts with him, but I remember conversing with her at length. She expressed a passion for teaching and research, and I sensed that she was a truly joyous and loving person. About halfway through our conversation, I also recognized that I was very attracted to her. But in the midst of a marriage going south, I didn't really give her a second thought when Sally and I left the party.

When I got divorced that summer, Steve called and asked if I wanted to drive with him and Candy to Chicago to see a Cubs game. As a lifelong baseball fan, I was about to say yes, until he said that Leah would be joining us as well. That sounded like a setup; and although I enjoyed chatting with her at the baby shower, I did not think it was a very good idea to be set up on a date with her. So I declined.

Later that fall, I drove my new Honda Accord from Purdue to Washington, DC, to attend our national convention. When I saw Leah entering a party, I immediately remembered her, especially when she beamed that engaging smile. I didn't know whether she was dating anyone, but I asked if she would be home on Thanksgiving, as I planned to visit my Polish grandmother on Chicago's south side. Leah said she would take me to her favorite nightclubs, but I wasn't sure if she was just being polite or flirtatious.

When I returned to Lafayette, I called her and we set a date for Thanksgiving Friday. And what a first date it was! When you live in Podunk, Indiana, Chicago is a very exciting city to play in. Leah took me to several bars, and after we closed down a blues club at 4:00 a.m., she invited me back to her place. We stopped off to get a six pack of beer—my first-ever St. Pauli Girl—and went back to her place.

We sat on her couch downstairs and chatted for a while. Although she was a smoker, which I thought was disgusting, I moved in to kiss her. She responded in kind, and we kissed for several minutes.

At one point, I twisted awkwardly, tweaking the chronic lower back pain I've had since playing baseball in college.

Leah asked if I was okay and then suggested that we go to a "more comfortable room" upstairs. She took my hand and led me to her bedroom.

I was so excited and so comfortable with her. Afterward, she lit up a smoke, which kind of killed the moment, but we talked until dawn.

I had told my grandmother, whom I called Naunny, that I would be out late, but I didn't expect to return to her house at 9:00 a.m. She and my Uncle Steve were eating breakfast in the kitchen when I stumbled in.

"Did you have a nice time?" Naunny asked innocently.

Before I could answer, Uncle Steve grumbled, "You better have had a good time since you were out all night with her."

I smiled, ate some high-cholesterol Polish kielbasa and eggs, and took a very long nap.

Two weeks later, I came back to Chicago to see Leah on my 28th birthday. She made a tasty shrimp dinner, and we went out all night long listening to music and dancing. I stayed the night again, which felt as exciting and comfortable as the first time.

When she asked me how old I was, she seemed shocked when I told her. I probably showed my surprise to learn she was 6 years older than me. But our age difference didn't bother me because I didn't expect our relationship to become serious. She smoked cigarettes, she lived in another city and state, and I was a young and recently divorced professor determined to make up for lost time after marrying so young.

Around this time, I dated a few women, some of whom were graduate students in my department at Purdue, although not in any of my classes. But I found myself thinking more about Leah and less about anyone else, except for one former grad student who had just left Purdue to teach part time at Northwestern.

I called the grad student and set a date for Friday of the Easter weekend. I also called Leah and arranged to see her the following night. I must admit to being very excited about the prospect of dating two women on consecutive nights in Chicago.

But then Leah called. She said she talked to the grad student and was not comfortable with me seeing both of them. I felt totally busted. I also was a bit upset when Leah essentially gave me an ultimatum to date her *or* the grad student.

I thought about Leah's position for several days. She told me she did the same thing the year before, and so I thought it hypocritical for her to take the opposite position now. But even though I wanted to see the graduate student, I liked Leah a lot and didn't want to mess that up. I called the graduate student and told her that I wouldn't be able to see her because I was dating Leah.

I could hear Leah smile when I called with the news. I still didn't expect our relationship to become really serious, but I wasn't ready to give up such a good thing just for one date with a former graduate student.

Leah showed up at our Hermosa Beach cottage much as I might have expected, in her Birkenstocks, old blue jeans, and an Iowa Hawkeye t-shirt. This was Leah casual—a bricolage of granola and corn fed. I knew better, of course. At Iowa, Leah had been my most challenging student. There was no slip of the tongue that Leah didn't leap to interrogate. Thinking aloud was at your own risk, cutting corners not allowed.

This was my wife Susan's first full dose of Leah. She didn't know what to make of this Leah book that didn't match its cover. And Leah didn't know what to make of this California thing. Sure Nick had told her. No sand and strand in Iowa. No skaters in bikinis. Bronze gods sure, but no doing a 360 on a beach break.

Leah took it in and giggled. It would take a while, but Leah's book was going to have a new chapter and a piece of the California dream. And it was all Nick's fault.

(Leah's former professor and their friend, Larry)

In May 1984, Nick decided to drive cross-country to attend the convention of our international association in San Francisco and to stay in California for a few weeks. His classes at Purdue were completed, but Northwestern was on the quarter system, and I would not be finished until June. However, I very much wanted to go to California—a place to which I had never been—and spend time with Nick.

He remained in California and then I joined him for 2 weeks. My friends took care of my dog, and Nick and I stayed with a college friend of mine in San Francisco for a week and did touristy things like ride the cable cars and go to Alcatraz Island. I hated San Francisco because it was cold and rainy, but I loved spending time with Nick.

Then we drove down Highway 1 along the Pacific Ocean. The ocean was so peaceful, awe-inspiring, and extraordinary, and I decided that someday I would live close to it.

I wanted to see Hearst Castle, and Nick suggested that we camp at nearby San Simeon State Beach. I had not camped since I was a little girl, but I was with Nick and trusted that he knew what he was doing. He parked the car and opened up the trunk, and I asked if he was getting a tent. He smiled and pulled out a single sleeping bag. We fit together very well in that sleeping bag.

The next day, we saw Hearst Castle and then drove to Los Angeles. We stayed a week with my friends, Larry and Susan, who lived a few houses from the ocean at Hermosa Beach. I loved L.A. because, although it was foggy in the morning, the sun always came out by 11:00 a.m. I could get up, have coffee and a cigarette, and walk on the beach. We went to see Disneyland, Dodger Stadium, the old Getty Museum, and Manhattan Beach, where Nick spent time as a kid with his cousins.

Nick and I also took a rather erotic shower together, the first time I had ever taken a shower with a man. It was awfully fun.

The 2 weeks just flew by, so much faster than I possibly could have imagined, and they convinced me that I was in love with Nick and wanted to spend the rest of my life with him. I remember thinking I sure hope he feels the same way.

I flew back to Evanston, and I did not hear from him that whole week. I was an emotional wreck. We had this most magical time, and I did not hear word one from him. I worried that I would never hear from him again.

I do not know where I get these insecurities. I guess they come from my first marriage and how that ended. I wanted to love and trust again, but I was afraid that I was going to be hurt again.

I went into a frenzy of home repairs to take my mind off my worries. I ripped up this ugly gold carpet that was in my townhouse on the main floor and on the stairs and refinished the wood floors. I painted my bedroom a kind of purple deep rose, and I painted the downstairs an off white because that made it look bigger.

Nick finally called me about a week later. I was so relieved. He is calling me, he did have a great time, he does like me. I remember the sense that the weight of the world had been taken off my shoulders. It was pure joy.

I taught summer school and then went home to see my mom. She had caught a cold that spring that turned into pneumonia. She could not get over it and became more and more tired. My dad took her to a specialist in Sioux Falls and then to the Mayo Clinic. They diagnosed her condition as congestive heart failure and determined that she had about 18% heart function.

I did not realize how serious her disease was until I called a friend who was a cardiologist. He said she maybe had 2 years to live. I was shocked. A heart transplant was a possibility, but she was a middle-aged woman, she would not be a top priority, and it would be very expensive.

I was still smoking cigarettes when I visited my mom. There she was struggling to breathe because her heart was not functioning, and there I was sneaking out back by the garage to have a cigarette. The dissonance was too great. I could not keep destroying my lungs while she was trying so hard to breathe through hers. I smoked my last cigarette on the final Thursday in August 1984 and never smoked a cigarette again.

I had been a two-pack-a-day smoker. I did not smoke two packs every day, but I lit two packs a day. I would take a puff and leave it in the ashtray and go do other things. Until I fought cancer, quitting smoking was the hardest thing I have ever done. That is an extraordinary addiction, and I did not realize how addicted I really was. I also did not have an appreciation of other people's addictions until that time.

When I came back and announced to Nick that I had quit smoking, he was very supportive. He came to Chicago for several weeks and that helped me keep my mind off of cigarettes. He was smoking a bit of marijuana, and he suggested that I smoke only to get high. Pot did help me quit smoking. Just that one little puff gave me the illusion of smoking, and it mellowed me out. It helped me go on for the next hour, then the next few hours, then the day, then several days, without smoking.

One of the things that Nick and I did that summer was to go to baseball games. We went to a bunch of games at Wrigley Field. We sat with the bleacher bums a lot because they were the only tickets we could get for some games. We also decided to write an article together about media coverage of the Cubs. It became more and more exciting during the season because the Cubbies did not fade. They hung in there and actually made the playoffs, although they fell one game short of making it to the World Series.

It was a glorious summer spending so much time with Nick. I knew I was in love with him, and I was pretty sure he was in love with me. Then school started, and Nick had to go back to Purdue, and we had to go back to a long-distance relationship.

I arrived at Purdue as a graduate student in the fall of 1984. Nick was an assistant professor in the Communication Department. Given how young he was, I suspect he felt more at home with the grad students than with the professors there. One day he told me that he was going to Chicago for the weekend to visit friends or family.

The following Monday, I asked him how the trip had gone.

"I had the best date of my life!" he exclaimed. And he told me about this wonderful woman he'd been set up with: Her name was Leah and she wore great hats.

I don't recall any more details, but I do remember to this day his glow! What a romantic way to begin a 20-year romance.

(Nick's friend, Patty)

I had a blast driving my Honda Accord cross-country, visiting friends and relatives along the way. But I was mostly excited to show Leah my home state of California.

I thought she would love San Francisco and hate Los Angeles, but the opposite was true. Of course, "the city" in the north had its typical cold summer fog, whereas "L.A." meant staying a few houses from the ocean in Hermosa Beach.

My favorite moment of the trip occurred at San Simeon State Park. When I asked Leah if she liked to camp, she said yes, although I didn't know at the time that she preferred "camping" at the Hyatt or Hilton. I don't know how she suppressed her shock when I pulled out one sleeping bag, but she took one look at it, one look at me, and smiled.

I suggested that we sleep on the beach, but it was too dark and deafening for a woman who had never heard the roar of the Pacific. We returned to the campsite and made love all night long under the stars. Thankfully, we made it to L.A. the next day and did not have to camp in that sleeping bag again.

I loved every moment of the trip with Leah, and I realized that I was falling in love with her. And I was not happy about it. I didn't think I was ready for love again, barely 1 year after divorcing Sally, and Leah still smoked cigarettes.

When Leah flew back to Illinois, I didn't call her for a while as I sorted through my feelings. I was supposed to be having fun in

California as a single guy with a new car, but I couldn't stop thinking about Leah.

I finally called her about a week later. She seemed a little upset, but mostly relieved. While talking with Leah, I decided to cut my trip by a week and return to Chicago to spend more time with her before school started.

I stayed with Leah and Rory Pooh at her townhouse for about a month. I was surprised to learn that this party girl who smoked, drank, and used marijuana on occasion attended church every Sunday. I was relieved when she wasn't upset that I didn't go to church with her.

When she returned to Evanston after visiting her mother, Leah announced that she had quit smoking. I said I was honored, assuming she had done this for me. She quickly corrected that she was quitting because of her mother.

I was happy Leah gave up cigarettes, but I was worried she would become moody and irritable as she suffered from withdrawals. Although she struggled at times, she controlled her emotions completely. She occasionally sniffed secondhand smoke at restaurants, which was gross, but she never lost her cool. I realized that if she were that calm while going through nicotine withdrawals, living with her would be easy.

The month in Evanston flew by, and I had to return to Purdue. The 2-hour distance that I found desirable in the beginning would now be a hassle. I wondered how long it would take before the commuting relationship became unreasonable and we would be ready for a change.

5

Life Changes

I was an undergraduate student in one of Leah's classes at Northwestern. She chewed a lot of gum and treated all the undergrads as grad students, so a lot of undergrads stayed away from her. But I liked her class and later became Leah's research assistant. I was her assistant when she ran the "Cherubs" program the summer when she and Nick were married. I ran the second video camera at the wedding and shot butterflies and other things for cutaways during editing, but I don't think we ever put together an edited version of the ceremony.

Leah treated you like an equal even though you weren't. She was the one who encouraged me to go to grad school, which I did. She was a very important person in my life.

(Leah's former student, Alex)

During the next year, Nick and I experienced more changes than we would in almost 20 years of marriage. Nick had been talking about getting a dog for several months, and in the fall of 1984 he finally did. We drove to a farm outside of Chicago, and he picked out a lovely little golden retriever that he named Wrigley. We came back to my townhouse and kept the puppy and Rory Pooh in the kitchen with a little gate.

That night Nick and I were in the bedroom when I heard a commotion down there and went to check. Nick woke up and asked where I was going.

I told him that I was going to the kitchen to make sure that Rory Pooh had not killed his new puppy.

Nick was a little panic stricken, not ever having lived with an Airedale terrier, but the dogs were fine.

That winter, Nick decided to accept a visiting professorship at Michigan State University for the winter and spring quarters. I helped him pack his stuff in Indiana and move into a cute little craftsman house in Lansing, Michigan.

Nick had sold his old sofa to his friends, Peggy and Paul, before his move, and so he did not have one. I said he could use this wicker couch and chair that I had on the patio for his living room furniture. One weekend I went to give some lectures at North Carolina State, and I brought Rory Pooh up to stay with Nick and Wrigley while I was gone. When I returned, Wrigley had done a nice little number on the couch, chewing off much of the wicker. It was not a 90-year-old antique couch, but I nonetheless was upset with him.

The drive from Chicago to Lansing would take 5 hours when the weather was nice, but we saw each other a lot and our relationship continued to grow. Rory Pooh and I would go to Michigan one weekend, and he and Wrigley would come to Chicago one weekend. It also was fun helping him to raise his new golden retriever.

That winter I was getting tired of all of the politics at Northwestern. I really liked Chicago, but I was ready to move someplace else. My colleagues, Lynn and John, had left Northwestern the year before to build a master's degree program at Southern Methodist University (SMU) in Dallas. That left me, a junior and still untenured professor, chairing a bunch of M.A., M.F.A., and Ph.D. committees and being the graduate director in the department. Lynn and John were a huge part of my support system, and they were recruiting me hard and heavy to join them and develop their graduate program. I was not sure whether I wanted to stay at Northwestern without them being there because everybody else seemed to be busy fighting about various things. It was not clear to me that there was going to be a lot of collegiality.

Nick had said to me ever since I first met him that he hated cold weather and that he did not intend to stay at Purdue more than 3–5 years. So I started talking to him about how I wanted to apply for other jobs and go someplace else. He was not really ready to leave Purdue, having been there for only 2^1/$_2$ years, but he was willing to explore other possibilities.

I remember going to a restaurant for lunch in Lansing in the early spring and discussing what we were going to do. Nick had somewhat reluctantly agreed to apply for jobs elsewhere, and we were discussing the possibility of him moving to Texas with me. I asked him if we would want to move as a married couple, and he said he was willing to move but not get married. That did not sound to me like a particularly convincing commitment, and I was worried that if things did not work out for him he would leave.

I told him I was uncomfortable with that scenario, and he reluctantly agreed to marry me. It was not an especially romantic engagement, but at least he had agreed to get married and move to Dallas with me if the jobs worked out, so I was very happy.

I applied for the job at SMU. They did not have a job for Nick, but they said they could create at least a part-time job for him in the business school and the communication department. Nick was a heavyweight scholar in communication, but he was not at all averse to being a communication professor in a management department. I interviewed for the job, and Nick flew down there with me to check on the possibilities for him and to look for houses.

Shortly after we returned, I received an offer from SMU, and Nick, in one of the most extraordinary acts of love and commitment I ever witnessed in my life, left being the golden boy at Purdue to go to a place where he did not have a tenure-track job to be with me. He once asked me if I would have done the same thing for him, and my honest answer is I really do not know. I was head over heels in love with Nick, and I wanted to marry him and spend the rest of my life with him, but some part of me really did not trust that a man would make that kind of commitment. I was not sure that if I gave up everything for my lover that my lover would be there and would not just leave me. But Nick was there for me, and he has been ever since.

That spring my mom's health continued to deteriorate, and I started to wonder whether she would be able to attend our wedding, which we planned for the summer.

Dear Leah and Nick,

We're so happy to hear the news of your engagement. We pray that the Lord will hold a bright and happy future for you to-gether as your plans begin to unfold. We love you very much.

All our love,
Mother and Dad

(*In a card from Leah's mother, Norma*)

Being a Los Angeles native, I have always rooted for the Dodgers. But when Leah and I studied how the media covered the Cubs in 1984, I also became a fan of the "lovable losers" of the north side. To our surprise, the Cubs won their division that season and were one game away from the World Series, a place they hadn't been since 1945. Then the Padres swept away our hopes in San Diego.

The day after the Cubs lost, the *Chicago Tribune* proclaimed, "PARADISE LOST!"

I read that headline and told Leah, "I'm going to get my dog today."

I wanted a dog for many years, but my first wife would not approve a pet until we were "settled," although we never seemed settled enough. When we divorced in 1983, I knew I would finally get my first dog as an adult.

Leah left her Airedale in her townhouse and joined me on the drive to a farm in Aurora. I inspected a litter of 8-week-old golden fluffballs, most of whom had massive paws, and Leah reminded me that Rory Pooh was a runt who might spend a lot of time playing with this big puppy.

I did not want a huge dog anyway, and the smallest male of the litter captured my attention. He cowered under a table as if his siblings had picked on him for 7 weeks and 6 days. I felt sorry for the little guy and brought him home. I named him after Wrigley Field, the friendly confines where the Cubbies play.

Wrigley was such a happy puppy. He loved curling up into a doggie ball on my massive beanbag chair in the living room. He moaned with contentment regularly, which was a bit embarrassing when he did so under the bed whenever Leah and I made love. At first we found it very distracting, but then it just became part of the experience.

Living with a dog was not the only change in my life. I took a visiting professor job that winter at Michigan State University in East Lansing. What had been a 2-hour drive from Purdue to Northwestern became a 5-hour drive.

Then on one visit to Michigan, Leah dropped the bomb that she was wanted to move to Dallas, where her former colleagues were recruiting her to teach. I knew I didn't want to stay in Indiana the rest of my life, but I wasn't ready to give up the best first job I could ever have, especially when she said there was no full-time position for me at SMU.

Leah and I had brunch at a restaurant in early spring and talked about our future together. I knew I was in love with her and was willing to explore other jobs, but I didn't want to give up my career for her. But I said I would consider moving to Texas.

Then she asked if we would move to Dallas as a married couple, and I told her I would prefer to go there unmarried, thinking I might need an escape hatch if things didn't work out. That was totally unacceptable to Leah.

I believed she would go there with or without me, and I considered the difference between a great job at Purdue without her and a not-so-great job at SMU with her. I decided the latter was a better choice. I told her I would marry her, and we ordered a glass of champagne to celebrate, although I had mixed feelings about it. I didn't sleep well for several days following that brunch.

Leah asked me to join her to meet her parents and to visit her sick mom. I was shocked when this big-city woman pulled into a tiny little Iowa town that seemed to be a life-sized Norman Rockwell painting.

Her mom and dad were cordial, but a bit cautious, probably because of my long hair and the earring I had implanted the summer before. Leah spent a lot of time with her mom, and it was clear she wasn't going to make it much longer.

My husband Paul and I met Nick when he taught at Purdue. We ran a Kinko's where he had his teaching materials printed. We became really good friends and hung out together a lot.

When he told us he and Leah were going to get married, he asked Paul and me to stand with him at the wedding as his "Best People." That was not very traditional and I had never done that, and I have not done it since. But extraordinary things happen when extraordinary people come into your life, and we were happy to be there with Nick and Leah.

Who could have known then that Nick and I would lose our spouses to cancer? I'll always remember when Nick and Leah came to visit us in Seattle before Paul died in 1992.

(Nick and Leah's friend, Peggy)

Nick and I were married on July 20, 1985, in the lovely Shakespeare Garden at Northwestern. Barb, my roommate in Iowa City, was my matron of honor, and Nick's friends, Peggy and Paul, stood up for him. My colleague, Lynn, and my student, Alex, videotaped the ceremony, although regrettably some construction work was occurring across the street so the audio was muffled by a jackhammer. After the ceremony, we went back to my townhouse for a champagne toast and then spent the rest of the afternoon picnicking and playing croquet and volleyball in a park in which we had reserved tables.

The day was bittersweet, however, because my mom could not attend due to her illness. My brother, Kevin, and his wife, Deb, came, but it was very sad that my mother's health was deteriorating so quickly.

Nick was not exactly pleased when I informed him that I could not go on a honeymoon because I was running the "Cherubs" program, a summer institute at Northwestern for college-bound high school students. I did not feel that I could leave these 40 rich kids that I was supervising. So the day after the wedding, I went back to the Cherubs, and Nick went back to Purdue for a few days to visit friends.

During the next few weeks, we packed up our belongings to get ready for the movers. I had worked one summer as a packer for a moving company, so I knew how to box up our belongings so nothing would be damaged. The day the packers arrived, I received a phone call from my dad. He told me that my mother had turned for the worse and that I needed to get home as quickly as possible. I flew home that day, but unfortunately my mom died while I was on the plane. She was only 55 years old.

A week or so later, Nick and I moved to Dallas and started teaching at SMU soon thereafter. That first year was a hugely hard year. It was so emotionally draining. I had a tenure-track position, but Nick only had a part-time job, and it was in a different area than he had taught at Purdue. He was not being treated like a tenure-track faculty member, and he did not know whether he even would have a job the next year. I would not have blamed him for saying screw this, this was not what I signed up for, and going back to Purdue. Although he was very unhappy, he did not say that and he did not do that. I used to think that I loved him more than he loved me, but I do not know if I would have stayed under similar circumstances.

At the end of that year, they finally opened up a tenure-track job for him, and life became a lot better. The next year, we bought our first house together, a Midwesterny two-story, four-bedroom one with a nice yard and a pool. We had a great life there.

One of my favorite memories is the party Nick threw for my 40th birthday. There were my university friends, my church friends, and other friends, and my dad, stepmom, and aunt came as well. It was like all the disparate parts of my life came together at once. We had Texas barbequed beef brisket. Nick put up pictures of me from different decades on posters, and people had to guess how old I was. It was really one of the loveliest birthdays that I can remember.

The next summer, we went on RAGBRAI (the Des Moines Register's Annual Great Bike Ride Across Iowa) across my entire home state with my dad, my stepmom, and her kids and their kids. That bicycle trip was probably our best vacation ever, although our butts were extremely sore and Nick had to get up very early in the morning each day. Nick also discovered that you can lean your expensive bicycles against the fence along with 7,000 other people in Iowa and it still will be there when you get back. He learned how to eat thick butterfly pork chops at 7:00 in the morning. It was quite an adventure and great fun.

I think the worst year of our marriage was 1988 to 1989, right after my 39th birthday. Up until that time, I had not really thought much about having children. Our attitude was that if we have kids it would be great, but if we did not have kids that would be okay, too. That year, however, a lot of people I knew who were close to my age were having children, and I started thinking that the future is now. I realized that I could no longer continue to think that maybe some day in the future I would like to have children because there are times when you have to say if it is going to happen it has to happen now. I started to think about what I would like to tell a child about my family and my upbringing. I thought it would be fun to nurture a little mind with all kinds of books, music, and interests. I also had the sense that I was alone in terms of certain aspects of my family lineage, and I wanted to pass that on. Nick also is great with animals and kids, so I approached him about it with my usual ox-plowing-through-the-doorway kind of approach. Needless to say, he did not respond well to that style.

We had many arguments about how we would raise this child in terms of school, religion, and discipline, but I think we ultimately would have negotiated those aspects quite well. I remember one of my positions was that any child who lived with me was going to have to go to church every Sunday until they left home, but that was not Nick's philosophy. After several months of discussion, however, Nick less than enthusiastically and wholeheartedly cooperated with me, and we tried to get pregnant over the course of 5 or 6 months.

I became really depressed when I did not get pregnant. I visited my OBGYN in Dallas, who suggested that we investigate a fertility clinic, but we had heard some negative things about those procedures and when I suggested exploring that option Nick he said no. I agonized over what to do about it for a long time. There were still a lot of positive things going on too, but the baby issue created a huge amount of tension, which was exacerbated when we did not get tenure at SMU and had to put our house up for sale and look for new jobs. After we settled into our new jobs and a new house in Sacramento, the stress from the baby showed up again and we had to go to counseling.

Apart from wanting to share things that were important to me with a child, I knew that Nick was younger than me. I worried that in 10 years he would change his mind about wanting a child and trade me in on a younger model. Counseling reassured me that would not happen. The counselor helped me to listen and really hear what Nick was saying, and he really was saying that he did not care if we had a child and he would not change his mind. I was still sad about not having a child, but I stopped being stressed about him changing his mind. I do believe that we would have been good parents. We certainly have been good dog parents.

I will always remember June 26, 1988. That was the day Nick and I beat Leah and another friend at Trivial Pursuit. Nick and I rolled the dice to see who would go first, we won the toss, and then we proceeded to answer every question until all of our pies were filled in. It was a perfect game! Leah and her partner didn't even get one turn.

I really enjoyed coming over to Leah and Nick's house in Texas on Sunday afternoons and playing croquet. I'll always remember Leah's smile and her hugs. She could kill you with a hug. You also couldn't get away with anything around her if it was indefensible. She would always challenge you, but never in a mean way. And she would make stiff drinks, especially after she gave up smoking. She said that was her one vice and she was going to enjoy it. I still make my gin and tonics strong in her memory.

(Leah and Nick's friend, Pat)

Our wedding day was a glorious one. The weather was perfect. Although our respective parents couldn't attend, many other friends and relatives shared the day with us. Everybody had a blast playing croquet and volleyball at the park.

Leah's colleague, Lynn, and student, Alex, shot video of the wedding, although when we replayed the raw footage from Alex's camera we mostly saw flowers and butterflies. He wanted those shots to make a more artistic video, although we never edited one.

I was not pleased when Leah told me she "couldn't" go on a honeymoon because of the summer institute she was supervising. I told her that she "wouldn't." I went to Purdue for a few days and hung out with friends, not exactly the romantic getaway I wanted. But I knew Leah's professional responsibilities would always outweigh her personal life.

The day the movers came to take our stuff to Texas, Leah received a call from her dad that her mom might not last much longer. Leah flew home immediately, and I stayed to complete the packing duties. I had to run a few errands and left Wrigley and Rory Pooh in the small backyard I had completely resodded a few days earlier. When I returned, they were caked with mud, having dug up most of the yard.

Later that day, Leah called me and said her mother died before she arrived. I drove to Iowa a couple days later for the funeral. I felt a bit awkward because I didn't know most of her friends and relatives, but I was there for Leah.

We returned to Evanston and stayed a few days in Leah's empty townhouse before we caravanned to Texas. I had the dogs in my Honda because her VW Rabbit didn't have air conditioning.

Leah was an early-morning person and I was a late-night person, so the long drive was a challenge. We hit the road earlier than I wanted but later than she would have preferred, and a few hours after sunset Leah was tired while I was still wide awake.

Around 10:00 that night, she signaled for me to pull over and said she couldn't go on. We stopped at a motel and snuck the dogs into our room. But Rory Pooh was restless and I couldn't sleep, so we agreed that I'd continue on the road with the dogs and we'd meet up at our rental house in Dallas. I lasted several hours before I parked at a rest stop to sleep for a few hours, but I still arrived in Dallas a couple hours before Leah.

Soon after we moved in, I read a magazine article in a supermarket line about various stressors in life that can affect mental health. Leah and I had just gone through almost every item on the list, including the death of a loved one, a change in jobs, a marriage, a new living arrangement, and a move. I figured if we could survive those stressors together, we'd be able to get through anything.

But I didn't expect my job at SMU to be so bad that first year. On my first day at the department, I met a professor who asked who I was. I said I was a new instructor who would be teaching public relations.

"Oh yeah," he said. "I heard Leah brought her boyfriend with her."

I had gone from a star at Purdue to the boyfriend who tagged along at SMU.

Apart from a bruised ego, the job turned out to be not what was promised. I was supposed to teach half time in the business school, but the chair of the communication department, without my consent, arranged for me to teach full time in his department teaching public relations, a subject I had only taught one unit on in one of my classes at Purdue. And it wasn't clear if I would even have a job the follow-ing year.

I was very stressed out for several months. I knew I had made a major career mistake. I wasn't sleeping well, and I'm sure I was irritable.

Leah's dad visited us for a few weeks in December. By then he was a widower of 5 months, and although he had met a woman, he seemed very lonely. I felt so sorry for him, and I wondered what it would be like to lose a spouse after so long.

The job situation became more positive the next year when the department created a tenure-track position for me. Leah and I also purchased our first home together, a four-bedroom, two-story one with a pool. We loved living there and quickly settled into a routine of work-ing, biking, swimming, and playing croquet. Life was great.

But on Leah's 39th birthday, she woke up before 6:00 a.m. as usual and tapped me on the shoulder. Very groggy, I somehow remembered it was her birthday and wished her a happy one. "I am 39 years old," she said. "If I do not have a baby by next year, I may never be able to have one. I need to have a baby this year."

Her announcement came as a complete shock. I was not opposed to having a child, but this wasn't the way I wanted the discussion to begin. I told her we could talk about it later and tried unsuccessfully to go back to sleep.

For the next several weeks, we discussed the idea of having a baby. We mostly argued about what this mythical child's life would be like in our home. We debated how long "she"—Leah had decided it would be a girl, and that her name would be Micah—would have to go to church. Leah demanded that Micah would go to church as long as she lived under our roof, whereas I insisted that once "*he* or *she*" was in high school they could decide for themselves. We also fought about other aspects of our childrearing philosophies without engaging in many childmaking activities.

We continued to quarrel for several months, and that summer I briefly considered moving out. But we continued to talk and ultimately recognized that we could work out the details of how to raise a child once we actually had a child.

We tried to get pregnant, but even that had its challenging mo-ments. One morning Leah woke me up very early after taking her temperature.

"Nick, wake up, I'm ovulating," she said. "We have to make love now."

I looked over at the clock. "It's 5:00 in the morning," I said. "Won't you still be ovulating in a few hours?"

Then we debated when we should have sex, instead of actually having sex.

After several months of trying, Leah did not get pregnant. Around this time, a friend told us about a couple she knew who also were trying to conceive. They paid thousands of dollars for fertilization, but it wasn't successful, and they nearly got divorced because of the stress.

Leah and I talked about their situation, and I said we could go through a similar experience with no guarantees. Leah said it was in God's hands anyway, which I took as an indication that she didn't want to pursue fertility options. We didn't talk about it again, neither of us was tested, and we continued trying to get pregnant on our own.

The year ended with two more challenges. First, Rory Pooh died suddenly of an aneurism at age 5. Leah and I were heart-broken, as was Wrigley, who started for the first time to sleep under the dining room table where Rory Pooh always rested. A few months later, we brought a new Airedale puppy into the household, whom Leah named Ragbrai after the Iowa bike ride.

Our second challenge occurred 1 week after Rory Pooh died when we learned that the SMU provost had denied us tenure after we received positive reviews from the department and the dean. We learned later that the provost had made a recommendation to the new university president to eliminate or downsize our department, so it wasn't surprising that she would reject jobs for life for two additional professors in that department. I'll never understand why the chair of our department didn't ask for our tenure reviews to be postponed a year until the decision on the department was made, as he knew about the provost's recommendation before our files went forward.

Leah and I stayed at SMU for our terminal year to finish a book we were coauthoring, but being there was awkward. Leah maintained her usual happy face at school, but she felt betrayed because she had been recruited to teach there. I actually was a little relieved because I didn't like living in Texas, and now we were forced to move.

In 1990, we accepted full-time positions at Sacramento State University and bought our first California home, which was half the square footage of our Dallas house, but twice the price. We enjoyed our jobs and camping on the coast with our dogs, but the stress of the baby issue unexpectedly resurfaced. On a few occasions, usually after drinking a bit too much wine, Leah described not getting pregnant as her "worst tragedy." The matter came to a head one night in the jacuzzi with some friends when, after all of us had drunk way too much wine, Leah blamed me for not getting her pregnant.

I was embarrassed because our friends heard this, but I was more upset that Leah was blaming me for not getting her pregnant when neither one of us had been tested because we were going to leave it in God's hands.

I was still angry the next day, and I told Leah that I would not tolerate being blamed for this. She apologized and suggested that we go to counseling. I agreed with her proposal for her to do a few sessions by herself and then a few sessions with me.

During counseling, I learned that Leah was afraid I might change my mind about wanting kids and leave her for a younger woman. I reassured her that I wanted to spend the rest of my life with her, not with anyone else. I also suggested that we adopt a child, but Leah wasn't interested in that option.

For the next dozen years, we enjoyed life together in Sacramento. Wrigley and Ragbrai died several years apart and, after grieving for each, we added Ebbet and Hawkeye to the family. We continued to teach, do research, and serve on committees, and we took day trips and camping trips with the boys. We traveled up and down the California coast, searching for a place to ultimately retire, and finally settled on Fort Bragg, where we bought eight acres of coastal property. We planned to teach 10 more years, build our dream house, and get old together. Everything was in place.

Then one day, while walking the dogs on the trail along the American River, Leah told me she had a stomach ache. . . .

6

The Shock of a Lifetime

To: kathy, mara, kimo, jan, peter, chuck, avery, gretchen, barker, beach, becker, berger, anne, bineham, bochner, dawn, browning, buzzanell, donal, clair, nickb, ccnrad, coopman, corman, ginger, amira, dion, dollar, drew, pedro, ellis, cellis, flanagin, frey, geist, goodall, gronbeck, josh, stacey, hafen, jani, stacy, ricky, heather, jenkins, kari, kidd, king, knapp, kreps, krizek, lamude, larson, wenner, wenshu, massi, may, thom, miller, chris, mills, motley, muto, neumann, asusan, billo, timi, putnam, roth, sanger, dean, shyles, smith, patty, candice, tmbo, bryan, jt, nikki, tracy, paaige, leah, vib, marlene, wall, williamson
From: nickt@csus.edu
Subject: Leah for WSCA VP
Date: 10/1/03

Hello Colleagues — For those of you who are members of the Western States Communication Association, you may have just received your materials and noticed that Leah Vande Berg is running for First Vice President. I would like to ask you to vote for Leah and to encourage other members of WSCA to vote for her as well. For those of you who are not members, I ask you to encourage department colleagues who are members to vote for Leah. Feel free to forward this email or send one of your own to other friends and colleagues around the country.

Thanks so much! Hope to see many of you in Miami for NCA and in Albuquerque for WSCA!

Take care,
nickt

After experiencing several days of abdominal pain in October 2003, I called my doctor and he advised me to go to the emergency room to have several tests run. I arrived in the early afternoon, and they started with a mammogram and an x-ray. They told me that I also needed a CT scan, but it would be $2^1/_2$ hours before they could do that because I had to drink barium before the procedure. Meanwhile, two nice young residents came in and performed a gynecological exam. At 6:00, they conducted the CT scan, my first CT scan ever. It felt very strange, like rolling into a giant tunnel.

About an hour later, one of the young residents came in and said that the CT scan was not positive. It showed some masses in my abdomen that were very suspicious and might be ovarian cancer. He said they were calling in a radiologist and a staff gynecologist to read the CT scan and do another exam.

I asked for some references to read and spent the next hour reading about ovarian cancer.

I called home and left Nick a message that I still was in emergency. I asked him to come to the hospital when he came home from class.

When Nick called, I told him, "Oh, Mr. Nickers, they think that I have cancer."

Nick arrived at the ER shortly after we talked, white as a ghost. About that time, the staff gynecologist, who had a Dutch name and piercing blue eyes, arrived and did yet another pelvic exam. He told us that he had talked to the radiologist and they thought I had Stage IV ovarian cancer. It appeared that tumors were in the abdomen, on the liver, and possibly surrounding the heart. The prognosis was not very good.

He prescribed medication for the pain and insisted that I take it because pain is hard on the body. He explained that the typical procedure was to have what they call a debulking surgery to get rid of as much of the cancer as possible and then to undergo chemotherapy. I asked about radiation, but he said they did not do that very often for ovarian cancer because it usually is not localized.

I was absolutely frozen in time as the doctor went over the diagnosis. It seemed like I was outside of my mind and my body and this was happening to someone else, except it very clearly was happening to me. It was such a grim and pessimistic diagnosis. I remember when the doctor said I had cancer, I said, "Hmm, that is very interesting."

Nick asked the doctor if it would be okay to go to the ocean that weekend, and he said, "If she were my wife, I would go tomorrow morning."

Nick and I went home and sat on the couch. We held each other and cuddled with the dogs. We both were devastated. Nick is much more expressive than me in many ways. He hugged me and cried. I was in too great of shock to be crying at that point. I took the pain pills and went to bed, although I did not sleep much at all.

It is difficult to express what I felt. I was not at all in denial. I recognized that it was not a diagnosis to argue with because I had been in pain and clearly something was seriously wrong. However, I was calm because I believed that God would take care of it and lift me up. I also fully believed that God could in fact choose to insert himself into this world that he created. Every day I began praying, "Dear God, please help me, please heal me, please forgive me, and please save me."

The next morning, for a moment, I thought it was all a bad dream. I only had to pat my tummy and feel how hard and distended it was to know that I was not dreaming.

I came into the kitchen and ate a light breakfast and took my pain pills. I read my devotions, which assured me that, no matter what, God was with me. The particular passages I read that morning are wonderfully enigmatic. Ask and it shall be given you, seek and you shall find. However, it does not say to actually ask for these things. I suppose one could ask for anything, and then God would be a tooth fairy and everyone would be a millionaire. Those passages gave me confidence that whatever God had in store for me, whether he would heal me or not, he would give me the strength to deal with it.

Nick loaded up our van and we drove to Fort Bragg. Nick called our friends, Cal and Susan, and they invited us to stay with them. Cal was the realtor who helped us find our land. Cal and Susan bought the lot that we decided not to buy and built a million-dollar home, and 1 year later we bought the lot they wanted to buy, but the owner would not sell to them at that time. Susan had been battling colon cancer for over a year, and I knew that she would be very supportive.

We arrived in Fort Bragg in the evening after the 4-hour drive from Sacramento. I sat down on the couch next to Susan, and she immediately put her arms around me and asked about my diagnosis. I drank a glass of Chardonnay, and we spent the rest of the night talking. They were wonderfully warm and encouraging.

The next day, Nick and I took several short walks along the beach. Every time I look at the ocean, this absolutely ineffable calming hand comes over me. I never feel far from God at the ocean. I experience a sense of being a little speck in the larger infinitude of creation. Stress and worry usually melt there. The ocean sweeps all of those cares away for me. It has done so ever since I first encountered it on a drive with Nick down Highway 1 in 1984.

The Fort Bragg coast was chilly that day. Nick and I held hands as we walked on the old haul road by our land. We went down to our little beach and threw sticks for the dogs.

The first time I cried was on our land. We sat in the van and looked at the place where we planned to build our house and bury our dogs' ashes, not my ashes. I had a few tears in my eyes before then, but that is when I really sobbed.

Although we could not afford to build the main house at that time, Nick suggested that we build a small guesthouse as soon as possible. We talked about the best-case scenario, that surgery and chemotherapy would be successful and my cancer would go into remission. We also talked about the worst-case scenario, that I would not survive the surgery. I told Nick I wanted to be cremated and scattered on the beach near our property and at my mother's grave in Iowa. I thought about and wrote down some of my favorite scriptures and hymns for the funeral. We talked about these things, by and large, in pretty calm ways.

Despite the circumstances, it was a joyous weekend.

Nick and I have never held a serious conversation. Instead we usually spend our time making fun of one another and when we get bored with that we make fun of the people that we know. But when he calls me about Leah I am absolutely floored. My grandmother died from cancer, a childhood friend is dying from cancer, and my mother in-law is battling cancer. I have never had a good experience with someone who has had cancer. Nick continues to explain what Miss Leah is facing. I remember merely responding O.K. after each thing that he tells me. I scramble to get a grip on what I am being told.

(Leah and Nick's friend and colleague, Kimo)

I first heard about Leah's cancer while sitting at my computer. It was 3:13 p.m., Friday, October 10th. The small envelope icon appeared at the bottom of my computer screen indicating that I had a new e-mail. My eyes were drawn to the subject line: Bad News.

It was not long after the start of the semester, and the last thing I was expecting to hear from Leah was that she had cancer. *I was stunned. My first instinct was to tell someone. My husband, Robert, is a man of few words, particularly when it comes to illness, and this news was no exception. The look on his face when I told him Leah had cancer spoke so clearly. His dark hazel eyes and long thick black lashes expressed the sadness, concern, and tragedy of a person who knows how devastating cancer can be. When he finally spoke his words were blatantly poetic, "That sucks."*

Robert was right. It did suck, and nothing could ease that bad feeling I had in my belly or lift the heavy fog that surrounded me when I thought about Leah having cancer.

(Leah and Nick's friend and former
graduate student, Jillian)

When Leah told me over the phone that she might have cancer, I felt like the wind was knocked out of me. I hung up, jumped into my 20-year-old Honda Accord, and sped to the hospital. I ran two red lights, although the hospital was 5 minutes away and it wasn't an emergency. I parked illegally in a doctor's spot and rushed into emergency.

I found Leah sitting up in bed, talking to a doctor with blonde hair and blue eyes. He introduced himself using a Dutch last name, and I smiled momentarily, knowing Leah would feel comfortable with a doctor who could have been from her small town. But my smile dissolved when his expression revealed how grave her situation was.

I hugged and kissed Leah. She wasn't crying and didn't even seem that upset. She nodded as the doctor detailed her condition and kept saying, "How interesting."

I reached over the rail of the hospital bed and clutched her hand.

"Oh Miss Leah," I said. "This is not interesting."

When the doctor told us that the cancer had metastasized to the liver and possibly the heart, time seemed to stop.

"That's bad, isn't it?" Leah asked.

"Yes, it's very bad," he said.

It sounded like an immediate death sentence.

The doctor left the room, and I looked at Leah. She smiled softly, and my eyes filled with tears. Calm as ever, Leah consoled me without crying, without showing any emotion whatsoever. She might have been in shock, but I attributed her reaction to her Calvinist upbringing—stoic, even at the moment she learns about her life-threatening disease.

I had an appointment the following Monday for a colonoscopy. Our friend, Susan, had developed colon cancer the year before and insisted that all her friends undergo the procedure. I was only 47 at the time, but she persuaded me not to wait until 50 because early detection can prevent the disease.

When the Dutch doctor returned, I asked if I should cancel my appointment and take Leah to the coast. He asked whether I had any rectal bleeding, and I told him no.

"If it was my wife, I would definitely cancel it," he said.

Leah insisted on driving "Little Red," her Honda del Sol convertible, back to our house, and I followed her. For most of the night, we sat on the couch, holding hands. I cried a bit more, and Leah again consoled me. When we finally went to bed, neither one of us slept much.

I lay in bed next to Leah in the dark with my eyes open, wondering what was going to happen to her. I rattled off a few silent Hail Marys, although I don't believe that God (or Mary) answers our prayers. To me, the only way the concept of free will can work is if God chooses *not* to intervene in human affairs. Otherwise he would be a Supreme Bureaucrat who spends his time processing several billion requests every day. Even so, repeating the Hail Mary ritual gave me comfort. And I thought that if anyone could heal a feminist with ovarian cancer, it would be a goddess.

Before we went to Fort Bragg the next morning, I called Cal and Susan to tell them about Leah's diagnosis. They invited us to stay with them.

I also posted a brief e-mail to inform people about the bad news. We knew that once word spread about her cancer, rumors would circulate, and we wanted our friends and relatives to have the most accurate information about her condition. I cued up the e-mail I sent to colleagues asking them to vote for Leah for vice president of our regional communication association, added another 20 or so friends and relatives, and sent word of her condition. Within minutes, a few friends called, although they didn't know what to say. They were in shock.

We arrived in Fort Bragg, and Cal and Susan greeted us warmly. Susan was hooked to an intravenous drip and appeared emaciated. I looked at her, saw Leah's future, and felt sick to my stomach.

I took Hawkeye for a walk to the beach to get some fresh air. I would have taken Ebbet too, but his front paw was injured.

Hawkeye and I made it to the haul road, and I knelt down and hugged him.

"It's you and me, Little Dog," I said and cried. "Leah's not going to be with us much longer."

He licked my chin.

We walked for about a mile in the pitch black. When we returned, Cal could tell I was distraught and gave me a glass of wine. Susan insisted that I take a sleeping pill, and I did so without hesitation and had a full night sleep. Leah refused to take a sleeping pill, worried that it would interact with her pain medication and the Chardonnay.

Early the next morning, Leah and I walked along the shore with the boys. I normally feel great solace there. The beach is one of very few places where I feel small but think big. I see the vastness of the sea and realize any problem on my mind is but a grain of sand in the cosmos. Instead of dwelling on personal concerns or office politics, I think about earth's place in the cosmos or about how the cosmos is reflected in a grain of sand.

But that morning I couldn't think of anything but the enormity of Leah's disease.

We spent the day doing what we typically do in Fort Bragg, but it was the least typical day we ever spent there. As usual, we walked on the haul road, played with the dogs on the beach, and enjoyed lunch at the North Coast Brewing Company, our favorite brewpub. But we had a most unusual conversation about her surgery, her possible death, her funeral, and her last wishes.

Leah was remarkably calm as she discussed these matters, until we visited our land.

"This *was* our dream," she said and wept. "I'm so sorry, Mr. Nickers."

We cried in each other's arms. Our plan to build a dream house and retire on the coast had been brutally shattered.

To: Leah list
From: nickt@csus.edu
Subject: bad news
Date: October 10, 2003
Hello All — Yesterday Leah was diagnosed with ovarian cancer that has spread to the abdomen, probably the liver, and possibly the heart. There are no early detection tests for this kind of cancer, and she simply had an upset stomach for

a few days that lingered on and motivated her to go in to have it checked. She will have another consult on Monday, followed by major surgery late next week or early the week after, followed by chemo, etc. She is at home for the next few days, though we might go to the coast for the weekend.

Our address is 4125 Bruhn Court, Sacramento, CA 95821; her e-mail address is vandeberglr@csus.edu

I'll let you know more when I know more on Monday.

Take care,

nick

I hear the news about Leah's cancer in a phone call from my fellow grad student, Jillian. I stop. Everything stops. I can't focus for a moment.

I ask, "What do you mean cancer? What kind of cancer?"

I need to sit down. Things will stop spinning if I just sit down. I am on the steps but I slowly sink to the floor.

I can hear Jillian's voice crack. I know that she is just as shocked and scared as I am. I don't know what to say. I'm crying.

I want to know everything. When is her surgery? What is the prognosis? How extensive is the cancer? How far has it spread? Where is she now? What do I do? How do I help?

I can't process this. I don't know what to think. Cancer equals death. Right?

I breathe. Finally. I breathe and I start hoping that she will be okay. I start chanting deep inside my soul, "she'll be okay, she'll be okay, she'll be okay."

I continue chanting. The constant hum of the words flows through me.

(Leah's former student and their friend, Juliane)

When I read Nick's e-mail about the "bad news," I only remember yelling, "FUCK!"

(Nick and Leah's friend, Thom)

When Nick and I returned from Fort Bragg, we were faced with many tasks to complete before my surgery. My first job was to call colleagues at school and ask them to take over my courses. I went to class on Tuesday and explained to my students that I had been diagnosed with ovarian cancer. I told them that I was having surgery, followed by chemotherapy, and would not be able to finish the semester. I assured them that the people who were taking over were thoroughly competent and they would be in good hands. I asked them to think carefully about the fact that life is short and about how they spend their time and how they treat other people. I told them that I was not afraid or worried because I had a very strong faith in God and whatever happened I knew that God would be there to take care of me. Some of my students cried. I did not cry, but I had a couple of tears in my eyes.

Nick accompanied me to the benefits office at school, where we met with an official about sick leave and disability. I had plenty of sick leave, enough for the entire academic year, but if I had to go on disability, then the university would no longer cover my insurance. Nick switched from his health plan to mine, so that if needed I could be covered on his plan and would not have to change doctors.

Nick and I met the doctor who would perform my surgery, a gentle man of Indian ancestry. He did his training at the University of Iowa, which I took to be a very good omen. When he walked into the examining room, he held out his hand, smiled, looked me straight in the eye, and said, "Dr. Vande Berg, I'm delighted to meet you." No physician had ever addressed me with that kind of respect for my academic title. It was the most caring, thoughtful thing he possibly could have said to me at that moment. I was absolutely blown away. He could have knocked me over with a feather.

We chatted about the University of Iowa and about Iowa City. He told us that his mother had died of ovarian cancer, so he knows very well the painful path of this disease. He spent over an hour with us. He down-graded my cancer to Stage III-C because no growths had penetrated the heart, and he was uncertain whether the detected spot on the liver actually was cancerous. He went over the CT scan with us on the computer in his office and talked about the treatments.

He had no trouble looking in our eyes, answering our questions directly, and making us feel that we were partners in the treatment. He explained that during the debulking procedure he would remove my uterus, ovaries, fallopian tubes, the omentum surrounding the intestines, and possibly part of the intestine depending on how much the cancer had spread. He said that you never know exactly what you are going to find until surgery, so it could take anywhere from 3 to 8 hours. If I made a little nonverbal wince when the news was bad, he would smile softly and place his hand on my knee.

My father and brother wanted to come to Sacramento because they were worried I might not survive the surgery. I was certain that I would survive, and I needed peace and quiet as well as time to absorb the physical, emotional, and spiritual shock. I also was in a good deal of discomfort because of the ascites, the liquid produced by the cancer, which had distended my abdomen. I asked them to visit on my birthday, a week after my scheduled surgery. They graciously accepted my wishes and let Nick and I spend this time together.

A few days before surgery, Nick took the boys and I on a day trip to one of the few covered bridges in the Sierra Nevada mountains near Bridgeport. I was unable to walk too far, but I could walk across the bridge with the doggies. The trees were starting to turn colors and were positively striking. The drive was very soothing because I could just look at the scenery and not worry about my cancer.

Nick was concerned because I had not cried about my situation except for the one time on our land. Part of me might have been in denial, but a larger part of me was absolutely convinced that I would survive surgery and that I was going to beat this disease. I did not feel that I should go around crying and feeling sorry for myself. I had a very positive attitude. Whatever happened, I knew that God would give me the grace to deal with it.

```
To: nickt@csus.edu, vandeberglr@csus.edu
Subject: Re: bad news
Date: 10/10/03
Dear Nick and Leah —
    I just got Nick's e-mail and I'm kind of in
shock. I can't begin to imagine how frightened you
both must be. I don't have a clue of what to say,
except that I love you both and I pray that you
get some better news next week. Please keep in
touch with me and let me know how you are doing.
    Much love and the best of wishes,
    Warren [friend and former student]
```

```
To: nickt@csus.edu, vandeberglr@csus.edu
Subject: Re: bad news
Date: 10/10/03
```

Leah and Nick,

I am so sorry for you, Leah. I will pray for you every single day for the next month. Prayers really do work wonders. I will pray for you Leah, Nick (that you can bear her pain), and for the dogs to continue to give Leah comfort....

One thing that is weird is that at my last "well woman" visit, the doctor didn't like something she felt and scheduled me for a sonogram. I have put off the appointment to have a biopsy until yesterday as well. So, Leah, your condition scares me for you, for Nick, and for me.

Love,

Mary [colleague and friend]

It seemed we had a million errands to run before Leah's surgery. I got substitutes for my classes the day of her appointment with the surgeon. He showed us the CT-scan, but it just looked like an impressionist painting on the computer screen. He said women in her condition lived an average of 3 to 5 years. The news wasn't good, but at least it wasn't the sudden death sentence we feared after the initial diagnosis.

We asked him to describe three possible scenarios from the best to the worst. The best case was the cancer would be isolated, surgery optimal, and treatment successful. The middle case was he'd find a lot of cancer, but surgery would go well, followed by chemotherapy. The worst case was he'd open her up, the cancer would be too widespread for surgery, and he would close her up and she would have months to live.

The surgeon was an excellent communicator. He answered the list of questions we brought with candor and kindness. We appreciated his directness, a quality we regarded highly throughout the process.

Leah's surgery was scheduled 6 days before her 54th birthday. In the meantime, we gathered as much information about ovarian cancer as we could find. I downloaded dozens of Internet sites and printed hundreds of pages and put them in a big binder. Leah's brother, a chiropractor and homeopathic specialist, sent us reams of material. We bought dozens of books as well.

We learned that ovarian cancer, like most cancer, is a horrible disease. Early detection of ovarian cancer is unlikely because it is not found with annual mammograms, pap smears, or blood tests. By the time a woman feels symptoms, such as abdominal pain or bloating, the cancer has already spread. The only test for it at the time of Leah's diagnosis was the CA-125, although the test wasn't reliable enough to be used in routine physicals unless there was a family history of ovarian or other gynecological cancers. Leah did not have such a family history, although her CA-125 levels were highly elevated.

When I returned to school, I started my first class by announcing my wife had cancer. A student cried and left the room. She later told me that her aunt was recently diagnosed with cancer. I informed subsequent classes about Leah's cancer at the *end* of the session. I told students I would probably miss other days during the semester, but I would find capable substitutes and class would continue regardless of what happened.

Every night leading up to surgery, Leah surrounded herself with so many pillows that she nearly sat upright in bed. She insisted on sleeping with Hawkeye, of course, but with him and the extra pillows, there wasn't much room in our antique brass double bed.

One night Hawkeye bumped into Leah's bloated stomach and she gasped. I told him to jump off the bed. He complied, but sat on the floor whimpering. Leah wanted to sleep with him, so she and Hawkeye went off to the guest bedroom. I objected because I wanted to be with her and hold her hand, but I realized where I stood in the pecking order of a dog lover's household. Leah's absence in bed made me toss and turn even more, and I wondered how soon I would be sleeping alone.

The next day we went shopping for a new bed. One of my students, whose mother had cancer, worked at a bed store, and he gave us a great deal on a queen-sized bed with dual controls. Leah could sleep on the soft mattress she preferred, and I could sleep on a firm one. More importantly, there would be enough room for Leah, Hawkeye, *and* me.

I didn't sleep much following Leah's diagnosis, maybe 3 hours each night, and I had nightmares. When I woke up every morning, I felt a fleeting moment of peace before the realization of her cancer jarred me back to reality.

I took a long shower to begin each day. I closed my eyes in meditative silence and let the water massage my back. Those 10 or so minutes provided a sanctuary in an otherwise stressful day.

I continued to send e-mail updates to Leah's many friends, relatives, and colleagues, and I asked people to forward the messages to others. One of my department colleagues told me that when his wife had cancer years earlier, he had to have the same conversation 20-30 times. With Leah's huge network of friends and family, calling people would have been a full-time job, so I e-mailed most of her friends and relatives.

These e-mails produced a bonanza of cards, flowers, and gifts. I strung up over 300 get-well and birthday cards underneath an archway in the living room, so every day Leah could see how many people were pulling for her.

A few days before her surgery, Leah wanted me to meet her pastors, Carol and Keith, from the Presbyterian church where she sang in the choir. As a mostly fallen Catholic, I attended services there on Christmas and Easter, but I didn't know the pastors personally. For the meeting, I wore my favorite tee shirt from the North Coast Brewing Company with the logo of their Rasputin stout. The front features a picture of the infamous Russian monk, along with Russian words that translate loosely as "Good friends take a long time to develop." I had adopted the shirt as my personal trademark because of the slogan on the back that reads "Never Say Die." I owned a few of those shirts and wore one almost every day, even to teach. Keith and Carol looked at my shirt several times during the meeting, and I wondered whether they thought the logo made some religious—or antireligious—commentary.

Leah and I spent much time sitting with each other and holding hands. We watched the baseball playoffs and were very excited when her beloved Cubs came within five outs of getting to the World Series. But then a fan interfered with outfielder Moises Alou as he tried to catch a foul ball, the team suffered a meltdown, and their curse continued.

Although I watched the games with Leah, I didn't really care about baseball that year. I just wanted my wife to survive surgery and overcome this disease.

7

Surgery and Recovery

```
To: Leah Update List
From: nickt@csus.edu
Subject: Leah Update
Date: 10/20/03
```

Hello All — Leah's surgery is tomorrow at 8:00 AM. She would love to see many of you before her surgery, but she knows that would be too emotional. So she's asked to see only her minister and her husband. (Her dad and brother will arrive Sunday so they can visit her in the hospital.) Thanks for understanding. I'll let you know when she's ready for visitors.

Surgery will take 3–7 hours. After surgery begins, I will probably hang out in the waiting room for a little while and then go home and wait by the phone. I live pretty close to the hospital, so the minute the call comes in I can rush over there and talk with the doctor.

Please have good thoughts, prayers, whatever works for you. I'll let you know what they find sometime tomorrow.

Thanks again for all your good wishes. I can't tell you what they mean to Leah.

Take care,

nick

Even with the pain pills, I was very uncomfortable during the week leading up to surgery. The ascites fluid was filling my abdomen, making my skin very tight, pushing against my organs, and causing a good deal of discomfort. Imagine having a pimple that is huge and ready to burst, but it just keeps getting bigger and bigger and keeps stretching the skin. The tumors also were pushing against my bladder, making me feel like I had to go to the bathroom multiple times each night, and it was a bit painful when I urinated.

I mostly was sleeping in the guest room with Hawkeye during this period. He always slept in our double bed with us, but I needed more room because of all the pillows that I used to prop me up. I did not want to sleep away from Nick, but I really wanted to cuddle Hawkeye.

The presurgery preparations were not much fun at all. I had to drink phospho-soda and take Dulcolax tablets to clear everything out of my system. I spent much of the day before surgery sitting on the toilet.

Between trips to the bathroom, I packed a light bag to take to the hospital. The surgical staff had given me instructions about what I could and could not take with me. I could not take glasses or my cell phone, and I could not wear any jewelry or watches. I took a sweater, pajamas, underwear, a couple books, and a little wire-haired fox terrier doll that a friend had given me that would be good to cuddle because I could not bring Hawkeye either.

I remember getting up very early the morning of surgery. I was not able to eat or drink anything. I did my usual morning devotions and I felt very calm. Although I knew there would be some pain from the surgery, I was happy that at last the discomfort from the ascites would be relieved.

We had to be at the hospital at 6:00 a.m. because I was scheduled to be the doctor's first surgery that morning. It still was dark outside when we arrived. A volunteer greeted us, and, after a brief wait, an admissions official called us into a small cubicle. She took basic information, including my religious affiliation. She suggested that I go to the bathroom one last time.

She led Nick and I and a few other patients to the presurgery area. I thought that I would get to stay longer with Nick, but we had to part at the door to preop. He kissed me goodbye and said he loved me and that he would see me in a few hours.

I was not nervous or at all worried. There was not a thing in the world that I could do at that point. I figured it was all in God's hands. I would not say that I eagerly anticipated the surgery, but I really was looking forward to getting relief from the pain. As I discovered, pain is incredibly exhausting for the body.

I calmly walked in following this nurse and another patient. The patient was a substantial woman, weighing about 250 pounds. The nurse put her on the scale and said, "Leah?"

I said, "No, I would be Leah."

She apologized and continued with our respective weigh-ins. She brought me to a room and told me to undress and put my clothes in a little bag. I put on a skimpy surgical gown and came back to the main room and lay down on a bed. I could see other people waiting for various preop procedures. The nurses came by several times and took my blood pressure and temperature. They asked whether I was cold and whether I wanted blankets, and they talked to me about the surgery.

The anesthesiologist came in and talked to me about the anesthetic. He explained the risks and said that they would start it in preop and I would be talking and then just slip away. I would not remember anything until I came out postop.

It was about a 7:45 a.m. when the nurse came over and said that the surgeon called from his cell phone to report that he was stuck in traffic. I would be his first surgery that morning.

About that time, Pastor Carol came into the room. She prayed, and the nurses prayed with her. I do not remember what exactly the prayer was. It was not a standard prayer.

Maybe 15 minutes later, the nurse came in with the anesthesiologist and said that the surgeon had arrived. She told Carol she would need to leave.

"We are going to give you some saline solution now," the anesthesiologist said.

Those were the last words I remember.

In my preop prayer, I usually thank God for the day, for the hospital and staff, and for medical arts. I ask that God give the surgeon discernment and that the patient awakens with the most minimal discomfort. No two prayers are alike because they are specific to the patient's situation. I prayed for Leah, and I prayed for Nick while he waited through the surgery. Silently I prayed for myself that I would be encouraging and affirming. It's hard to say this, but sometimes I "just have a feeling" about some people—whether they will recover or not—and I had a feeling about Leah. It was not good. I do not want to transfer this feeling to the patient, and I really want to be wrong, but seldom am.

(Leah's pastor, Carol)

I slept for maybe 2 or 3 hours the night before Leah's surgery, but I was wide awake when my alarm went off at 5:00 a.m. I fed the dogs and took them outside before we left for the hospital.

When I kissed Leah goodbye in the hallway near the preop area, I honestly wondered whether I would ever see her again. Unlike Leah, I was worried that she might not survive surgery. Neither of us had ever gone through a major operation, and this procedure seemed as major as it could get.

The surgeon told me to stay in the waiting room for about a half hour in case anything went wrong immediately, but then to go home and wait for his call. He said surgery could last up to 7 hours.

On the drive home, I prayed. "Dear God," I said, "if you're going to take her anyway, take her now rather than make her have a long painful death."

I flashed on a M*A*S*H episode in which Hawkeye has a patient who needs an organ transplant and B.J. has another patient who he can't save, so they're waiting for him to die to be the donor. In one scene, Father Mulcahy tells God he never asked him to take someone's life, but if he was going to take the patient anyway to take him quickly so they could save the other one. I felt just as conflicted. How could I possibly ask God to let my wife die during surgery? Easy, if the alternative was a slow painful death.

In fact, dying in surgery seemed to be the *second* least desirable result. The most ominous outcome was finding so much cancer that they couldn't operate, and Leah would have a few weeks to live before a possibly excruciating death. I was tormented, imagining her various death scenarios.

When I arrived home, I immediately played two recordings that had become theme songs. The first was Tom Petty's "I Won't Back Down"; the second was Sonny Terry and Brownie McGhee's "Jesus Gonna Make it Alright," written by M. Franks. I played them over and over and sang them loudly. Even in my sleep-deprived state, I recognized the irony of a fallen Catholic singing about not backing down at the gates of hell and hoping that Jesus will make it all right.

After singing to exhaustion, I sat down on the floor in the living room and cuddled Ebbie and Hawkeye. Ebbet always has been very sensitive to the emotions of his human companions, and when I cried he pulled himself away from my hug and went to the back bedroom.

"Thanks for your support, Ebbet," I said and laughed momentarily.

Hawkeye stayed very close to me.

My adrenaline started to wear off, and I went to the bedroom to take a nap. I placed the phone on a nightstand next to my bed so I could immediately answer the call from the hospital. I had just fallen asleep when the phone rang. I jumped up, thinking it was the surgeon, but it was our neighbor asking how surgery went. She could tell that she woke me up and apologized. I told her I would call her as soon as I knew something.

I lay back down and minutes later the phone rang again. I jumped up and repeated the conversation, this time with a friend from out of town. He apologized and hung up, but then he accidentally called me back and asked for John. When he realized he had dialed the wrong number, he hung up.

About an hour later, the doctor called. I was concerned that he called after just 2 hours in surgery, but he assured me the operation was very successful. I told him I would be at the hospital in 5 minutes to get the full report.

I paced in the waiting room until the surgeon arrived. He said he had good news and bad news. That is a line you want to hear in a joke, not about your wife's major surgery. The good news was that surgery was successful, an "optimal debulking," as he described it. He removed most of the cancer and did not have to cut off any of her intestines. He was unable to remove the lesion on her liver, but he still wasn't convinced it was cancerous.

The bad news was that Leah had the worst kind of cancer: carcinosarcoma or malignant mixed mesodermal tumor. He called it the most aggressive type of cancer; although they cut most of it from her body, it was certain to grow back.

He said Leah wouldn't be admitted to a room for a few hours. I went home and sent an e-mail about her surgery and called a few relatives who did not use e-mail. I returned an hour later and sat in a small waiting room on the wing where Leah would spend her recovery.

While I waited, I met a man in his late 50s or early 60s whose wife also had surgery for ovarian cancer that day. I asked how he was holding up and he started to cry. I hugged him for a couple minutes, and then we talked about her situation. He said his wife's doctor had not told them anything about her condition, and I was surprised to learn that she and Leah had the same surgeon. He told me they met with him a week earlier, but they didn't know what to ask. I was relieved that we brought a list of questions to our appointment with him and we insisted that he answer our questions directly.

Pastor Carol joined me in the waiting room, although I don't remember what we talked about. After an hour or so, I asked a nurse when Leah would be admitted. She said they were ready to check her into one room, but an elderly woman patient in that room was too noisy and they were waiting for a more quiet room to open up.

They finally wheeled Leah into the room. She was very groggy, but managed to open her eyes. She looked at me and I smiled.

"Yes, he's smiling," Pastor Carol said.

"How is the liver?" Leah asked.

I was amazed she was cognizant enough to ask about her liver. I told her it was fine, not wanting to give her the specifics. Overall, the surgery was good news, and I wanted to be completely positive at that moment.

I stayed with her for about an hour, but she faded in and out of consciousness. I went home and collapsed on the floor, absolutely drained of energy and about ready to lose it. At that moment, Ebbet walked over and dropped a toy right on my face. "Play with me," he whimpered with a wagging tail. I started laughing and played tug of war with him and Hawkeye. I realized I might have had a hard day at the hospital, but the boys were waiting all day for me to come home and play with them.

To: nickt@csus.edu, vandegerlr@csus.edu
From: Michael
Subject: Best Wishes
Date: 10/14/03
Nick & Leah —

I was so sorry to hear the news. I'll be praying that the surgery goes well — that they get it all, that the metastasis biopsies and tests are negative, and that the recovery is rapid.

Even with the best-case scenario, this damn disease plays some horrible games with the mind, and sometimes the body; and of course even more so under the less favorable scenarios. Here's hoping for a best-case scenario, and for many more good days than bad days in any case.

I'm not going to do the "I've been there" bit except to say that I'll be calling from time to time, and if either of you ever wants to ask me ANYTHING about my wife's and my experience, please DO. Of course, if there is any other way I can help, let me know; but especially I want you to know that I'm glad to talk about any aspect of my wife's ordeal, or mine, if it will help either of you even a little.

    Best wishes on the surgery. I hope — and will continue to pray — that they can get it all and find that it hasn't spread.

    Love to you both,

    Michael (friend, whose wife died of breast cancer)

I have a vague memory of moving and trying to sit up after surgery, but it is really cloudy. The next thing I remember is being in a hospital room. Nick was there, and I think Carol and the surgeon might have been there, too. I do remember Nick holding my hand and leaning over me and saying it was okay. I think the doctor told me that it was an optimal surgery and that my liver was fine.

I floated in and out of consciousness for a longish time. I do not know how long I slept. Nick was there sitting at my side. I was in some pain, and I had all kinds of tubes hooked up to me. The nurse came in and checked on me periodically. There were flowers everywhere. I remember Nick saying goodnight and that he would be back in the morning.

My half of the room was very small, and I had an IV hooked into me from stands on both sides of the bed. I also was hooked up to a catheter as well as another tube in my abdominal cavity that was draining out ascites and blood and goop. They had to empty that bag every few hours. I also was hooked up to another machine that alternately squeezed and released my calves because my legs were swollen from edema. I felt like I had elephant legs.

On the morning of the second day, the nurse came in and said, "Okay, you have to start walking now."

I remember laughing and thinking, Right, I have a huge incision from my belly button to my vagina, and I have to start walking?

She said that she was not kidding and that I would have to walk several times a day in the hallway. She explained that the sooner I started walking, the sooner I would get my fluids going and the sooner my bowels and urinary track would start moving. As soon as I passed gas or had a bowel movement, I would be able to go home.

Walking was exceedingly difficult and painful at first. The nurse had to unhook my legs and swing me around and then roll my IV stands together. Initially somebody needed to walk with me because I did not have any balance and I could not yet push both of the IV stands while I walked.

Each morning the nurses would get me up and serve oatmeal and a little juice. Then I would sit in a chair and read my devotions and various books and magazines that visitors brought. I could not get up to push the button above the bed to call the nurses. After I became stuck there, I subsequently brought all of my books to read while I waited for the nurses.

On the second or third night, both IV machines and the calf exerciser stopped working. The young nurse who was on duty could not figure out what was wrong with them, and they just kept beeping and beeping. This went on for about 45 minutes. My head was ringing, and I was pretty grouchy. I asked for a nursing supervisor to come in. She took a long time to arrive, but when she did she took one look at each of them, went click, and bingo, the noises stopped and the machines started working again.

By the third day, they took the catheter out, which meant I had the challenge of going to the bathroom. I had to call for a nurse, and they did not always come right away. That would be an understatement. They had to swing my IVs around and help me walk to the bathroom. Then they would have to wait and help me move them back. Fortunately, I still had good upper body strength, and I was able to hold my body up above the bed while the nurse would swing my leg up and over onto the bed so I could lay down.

On day 3 or 4, the bag that was draining the blood and the postsurgical fluid was full. I rang for a nurse and eventually he came, and I told him the bag needed to be emptied. He picked it up and started shaking it to get the air bubbles out. I said I did not think that was such a swell idea because it was pretty full, but he insisted that he always did that before taking it off. Of course, it burst open and spewed blood and cancerous fluid all over me. He had to clean me up, change the sheets, and mop the floor.

I thought that the surgical staff was amazingly attentive, but the ward nursing staff was abysmal. There were some really caring and compassionate nurses, but I never knew from one shift to another whether I would have a knowledgeable competent nurse or someone who absolutely did not have a clue and who probably did not do well in nursing school. Some of the nurses did not even know anything about my case. As a result, right after surgery and when you are in pain and tired, you, the patient, have to make sure that you tell them what is going on with you and what you need to have done. You need to monitor that you are getting the meds you are supposed to be getting, and that the bags attached to you are emptied appropriately. I found that to be very frustrating.

The food they prepared was awful. The jello, soup, and everything else I ate seemed to be red or yellow, the color of blood or urine. I begged to have mashed potatoes, but they would not give me mashed potatoes.

My doctors came by every morning, and by day 4 they started asking me whether I had passed gas yet. I said no, but I was walking in the morning, the afternoon, and the evening to get my system to start functioning again. I tried to do everything I could to pass gas and go home so I would not have to stay on that little ward of horrors much longer.

Many friends and colleagues came to visit. Pastor Carol came most days. My graduate students brought me a panoramic picture of all of us at a birthday party a month before. Other colleagues brought me haiku books and mysteries and magazines. It was tiring but wonderful to have lots of folks visit because sitting in there was kind of lonely. It was nice to know that people cared enough to take time out of their busy days to come over and see me.

Nick was there every minute that he possibly could be. He would regularly come to see me two or three times a day, even on his long days on Tuesdays and Thursdays. He was teaching his classes, feeding the dogs, taking care of the house, and trying to get a little sleep. He got hugely worn down. But every night he was there, holding my hand while we watched the World Series.

The room was so stark and antiseptic with white walls and no paintings to make you think about getting well. Fortunately, my relatives, friends, and colleagues were flooding me with cards and flowers, which were hugely appreciated and made the room much more cheery. Nick also brought in photographs of the ocean and of the dogs and I to brighten it up. That was wonderful, a very homey touch; however, I also wanted one of Nick so I could see him when he was not there. I reminisced about all the fun we had walking on the beach. I thought, I am going to beat this disease and walk on the beach for many more days.

I kept receiving many bouquets of flowers from people all over the country. My relatives, friends, and colleagues were flooding me with cards, and that was very sweet and touching. Every day Nick would bring some flowers home because I would get a new batch. The flowers were beautiful and made the room much more cheery.

My dad and my brother arrived a couple days before my birthday. They had not seen me all swelled up and sick, and I think it was a bit of a shock to their system to see me like that. I am sure it was déjà vu all over again for them, having seen my mother in the hospital bed. They were great about coming over to visit for a little while and then going and letting me rest and then coming back.

One night after my dad and my brother came to visit, they went with Nick to eat at a restaurant. They came back with a little cache of mashed potatoes for me. Unfortunately, I could not eat them because a new nurse gave me a different sedative that night. By then I always asked what they were giving me, and this nurse said he was going to give me one that I had not taken before. I told him that I wanted the other one that I had been getting, but he said my doctor had authorized three sedatives and he gave me the one I did not want intravenously. I became very dizzy and incoherent. I called for another nurse to come in and explained what happened, and they gave me some fluids to try to flush it out of my system faster. Shortly thereafter, my dad and brother and Nick arrived from dinner with the mashed potatoes, but I was out of it. The nurse said it would pass through my system quickly and that I should sleep it off. I did, but it was not until four in the morning that I finally fell asleep.

Nick told us that Leah was getting restless in the hospital and visitors were welcome. I could think of no better way of brightening Leah's spirits than bringing her some of the most heavenly chocolate cookies from a French bakery not far from the hospital.

Leah was resting when I arrived, but rallied to welcome me. Leah looked like Leah, except her legs were swollen. We talked about the appallingly uninteresting walls of her hospital room, baseball, and the crappy hospital food. Little did I know that all Leah could eat was broth. What a fool I was for thinking that a woman who just had a radical surgical procedure in her abdomen could eat freakin' chocolate cookies.

Leah was courteous when she declined my offer of a little piece of chocolate comfort. I could see Leah's energy was beginning to fade, so I hugged her goodbye and sheepishly left with my cookies.

(Leah and Nick's friend and former graduate student, Jillian)

To: Leah Update List
From: nickt@csus.edu
Subject: Leah Update
Date: 10/22/03
    Hello Again — Leah had a tough night, but that's to be expected following such a surgery. She'll be in the hospital for 5-10 days, then come home for recovery and a long treatment process.

As fate would have it, she'll very likely be in
the hospital for her birthday (Oct. 27). Cards
and flowers have been and will continue to be very
much appreciated. For those who know her well
enough to send gifts, BOOKS would be great at
this time, since she'll be spending a lot of time
in bed. She loves mysteries with female sleuths
written by women — the problem is that she has
virtually everything Agatha Christy, Amanda Cross,
Dorothy Sayers, Carolyn Hart, Margaret Truman,
and Antonio Frasier have written, but that's
the type of mystery she likes. (No thrillers.)
Being the feminist, she likes virtually anything
about feminism/women's studies, and also likes
biographies, preferably about women....

   Thanks for your kind words and offers of
support, not only for Leah but also for me. I
have indeed had some sleepless nights and have not
been exercising regularly, but I know that I need
to pay attention to my health and well-being too.
I appreciate all of you friends and colleagues.

   Thanks also for your positive responses to
these e-mails. I've never appreciated the power of
e-mail more than at this time. It has been a way
of keeping in touch with MANY people, and even
though I haven't been responding to individual
e-mails, I really appreciate your replies.

   I'll be stopping the regular e-mails at this
time, and just let you know when she comes home
from the hospital. After that, I'll just send
monthly/quarterly updates on her condition.

   Take care,
   Nick

Leah's postsurgery recovery period was very challenging. Her room was
very small, probably 10 feet wide and 15 feet long, and there were two
beds. Leah was crammed in the end of the room, very close to the
wall. The walls were colorless, a dingy off-white color with no pictures
or paintings.

   I should have insisted on a bigger room, but I had just endured
my wife's surgery and wasn't thinking about the room. I was so

thankful she had survived surgery that I didn't even think about the postsurgical situation.

A bad omen occurred the first day. Leah was hooked up to four machines: two IVs, a catheter for the urine, and a machine to stimulate the calves because of the fluid in her legs. I had been there for about 15 minutes when the stimulator stopped working and started to beep. I didn't know what this machine was, so I went to retrieve a nurse. I found one and she said they had been having a problem with the machine. She fumbled with buttons, but nothing seemed to work. Then she clenched her fist and smacked it, and it started to work again. I admit I have kicked the tires of a stalled vehicle, but I was not in favor of the same approach to a machine hooked up to my wife.

I was appalled when on that first day I saw sick feeble women dragging IV machines on wheels down the hallways. The day after her surgery, Leah became one of those women. I learned that walking is essential to recovery, but it seemed cruel to make women who had just had major surgery drag their two IV machines down the hallway. I walked with Leah each day, at first halfway down the hall and then all the way to the maternity ward, although she was not allowed to go to the viewing area to see the babies.

Leah and I watched the playoffs and World Series each night in her room. I visited her at least twice a day and often three or four times. Fortunately, it was just a few miles from our house, a 5-minute drive when there wasn't traffic.

One night the IV machine started to beep and yet another nurse couldn't figure out how to fix it. She put in new batteries, but it still wouldn't work. She said she was going to get help, but then disappeared for about 30 minutes. Finally, a different nurse came and determined that a little clamp was preventing the IV solution from entering the veins.

About 30 minutes later, Leah said she had to go to the bathroom, but the nurse insisted that she had a catheter and should not feel any discomfort. I insisted that she check it, and she found the plastic tube to the bag pushed so far under the bed because of the cramped space that it prevented Leah's urine from feeding into the bag. The nurse pulled it out and Leah felt immediate relief.

About 15 minutes later, the other IV machine stopped working. A new nurse put in another IV bag, and then blood appeared in the tube. The nurse insisted that was a good sign, but it had not happened before and did not seem to us to be a good sign.

Leah was very distressed about the malfunctions of the machines and the apparent incompetence of some of the nurses. I got angry as well and yelled at one of the nurses. I thought the malfunction of all four machines was simply unacceptable. That night I wrote a letter of complaint to the Chief of Staff, although I never received a reply.

I e-mailed a colleague who specializes in health communication and runs a health communication institute. She replied that our experience was typical of health care in America. I felt total frustration and complete powerlessness.

But these experiences did make me more assertive in subsequent interactions with the nurses, and they led me to take a more active role in Leah's care. Whenever the IV malfunctioned again, I adjusted the little plastic shutoff valve. I smacked the calf machine myself when it stopped working. I pulled the catheter bag to keep the fluid coming. I probably violated hospital policy doing these things myself, but at least they were getting done.

I printed off and taped up a few photos of the ocean in Fort Bragg to add color to the room. I also put up a picture of Leah and the dogs from when she was not sick. Leah didn't tell me she wanted one of me until her last day there.

Leah received so many vases of flowers that there wasn't enough space in the room to keep them. Whenever I walked the halls to get to Leah's room, I always noticed rooms with older women that had no flowers or visitors, and I asked a nurse whether I could give some of Leah's flowers to them. But she told me it was against hospital regulations to put flowers in rooms unless you are a family member. I should have violated that policy too and distribute vases to various rooms, but I just took them home until they became too musty.

Although Leah wanted the Cubs to get into the World Series, she was happy when the Florida Marlins beat the Yankees. She would have been happy to see the Yankees get beat by anybody.

Her dad and brother arrived a few days before her birthday. One night I came home from school and her brother said I needed to go to the hospital because Leah was upset that they had changed her drugs.

I rushed over and discovered that a new nurse had given her a different sedative than she was used to receiving, and she was more groggy than usual. She was very upset because she wanted to be more alert during her dad and brother's visit. She was mumbling and not very lucid.

I held Leah's hand and calmed her down. I told her I would tell the nurse to always give her the other pain medication, and she would have a nice visit with her dad and brother tomorrow. I held her hand until she fell asleep.

Even with regular visits from family and friends, Leah felt very lonely at the hospital. And she experienced an almost complete sense of powerlessness, which was especially upsetting because Leah was a bit of a control freak.

I'm sure that was one of the longest weeks of her life.

I had spent the days leading up to Leah's surgery thinking of a gift to buy her. I notice that Miss Leah does not wear a cross necklace, but I know that she is very religious. While she is in surgery I go shopping by myself in jewelry stores to find a cross necklace for her. I find something that I think is perfect for her that is simple and elegant.

I give it to her in the hospital. She opens it up and immediately puts it around her neck. We are alone in the room and I comment on the number of flowers she has in her room. She is amazed by the graciousness of others. We talk about the book that she is reading, laugh about hospital food, and make fun of Nick. Even during the worst of times we could always find ways to have fun laughing at Nick's expense.

I was deeply touched by Leah. I never saw her again without wearing the cross necklace that I gave her. My wife now wears Miss Leah's cross necklace. I think of her every time I see it.

(Leah and Nick's friend and colleague, Kimo)

The day before my birthday, I was walking down the hallway and I passed gas. I exclaimed, "Yes!" I was never so excited to pass gas in my lifetime. Although I was a little afraid to go home because of my sutures, I was very eager to leave that little ward of horrors.

The next morning, the surgeon came by and said, "You're going to get to go home today." He answered my questions about what I needed to do at home. The nurses came by with all kinds of paperwork and information about my medications.

They also had to take out the little bag that was draining fluid out of my abdomen. The nurse said, "This is going to hurt a little bit," and he took it in his hand and yanked it out.

It hurt badly, and I was gasping for breath.

I said, "That didn't hurt a little bit, it hurt like hell."

He apologized, but he had been in the military and I guess this was not a big deal from his perspective. They patched up the hole about the size of a straw and I was ready.

I was so delighted to be able to go home on my birthday. My colleague, Sylvia, happened to be visiting that day, and she helped me get dressed while Nick went home to get the Monster van. The van was easier to get into than the Subaru because of the higher front seat. My dad and brother took a bunch of my cards and flowers.

When we arrived home, I settled in on the couch and immediately Hawkeye jumped up and cuddled on my legs. My little companion dog was so happy to see me.

Nick made me a birthday dinner of salmon, broccoli, and mashed potatoes. I even sat at the table to eat it. I was home on my birthday with my family. It was wonderful. I said, "Thank you good and gracious God. Thank you for this glorious day!"

Nick showed me the bed that had arrived while I was in the hospital, a beautiful new adjustable bed that I slept in that night for the first time. The bed was really great because it is really high, so I could just lean back and sit on the bed and push myself back a little bit and swing my legs over. I did not have to pull myself up to get in or push myself down to get out.

Unfortunately, our national convention came up about this time, and there was no way I was in any kind of shape to fly to Miami, where it was to be held. Nick did not want to go by himself and leave me here, so we cancelled our trip. That is one of my regrets about the timing of the surgery. Some of our friends called us from the convention to let us know that they wished we were there partying with them.

I ate pretty regularly and regular kinds of foods. The doctors said that if my bowels and urinary tract were working and everything kept moving through, I could eat whatever I wanted. I had done a bit of reading about ovarian cancer, and I learned that it is better to eat a low-sugar and low-fat diet. We had a pretty good diet to begin with, mostly fresh fish, chicken, vegetarian dishes, and a lot of green leafy vegetables, which are supposed to be good anticancer foods. We had largely cut out cheese except for feta, which is lower in fat. For the last year and a half, we also had been eating mostly organic foods.

My dad and brother left the day after I came home. I was very happy they had come to see me, and I think that they were reassured that I would recover from surgery.

A few days later, my good friend, Laurie, who is a thyroid cancer survivor, came to visit. She was a geologist for an oil company and lived in Alaska at the time. She was traveling in the lower 48 states for a meeting, and she rerouted herself back through Sacramento and stayed for a few days before flying back to Alaska. She is such a wonderfully adaptable low-key guest. We just sat around and talked, watched some TV, did crossword puzzles, and made food. We also took a short day trip to the foothills.

When Laurie left, Nick's mom, Claudia, came for a visit. Claudia is somewhere between a big sister, a friend, and a mother figure, and we get along splendidly. When we first met, we smoked cigarettes and drank wine together. Then I quit smoking and 10 years later she quit smoking, but we still drank wine.

Nick and I had asked Claudia to come to help me, but it turned out that I really did not need any help as long as I did not try to lift anything heavy. I was far more ambulatory than we initially had expected when she agreed to visit. We did go grocery shopping, and we made a little foray to the mall, but I did not require her help to go to the bathroom or bathe.

Claudia has a very different style of intimate relating than Nick. She has a need for verbal intimacy. Except for those times when she is doing her religious readings or meditating in the morning, she needs to talk to people. She and I have been known to have 3-hour conversations on the telephone. We can just talk and argue—not fight argue, just take different sides on an issue. I loved having her there and talking to her.

Nick, however, has a very different style of relating. He and I can take a drive and sit in absolute companionable silence for a goodly length of time. At night, we will often sit in the living room grading papers or writing with the TV on in the background, and that is just fine with us. Although we talk to each other very openly, we also can express intimacy through being in the other person's same space without verbally expressing ourselves. I sometimes very fondly call him a "hermit crab" because he is perfectly happy to retreat into his study and work, emerging only to eat or walk with the dogs or have an occasional tennis or golf game with Kimo.

Nick usually is a wonderfully gracious host, but he was exhausted from teaching his classes and coming home and dealing with the dogs and cleaning the house for all of these guests. He had reached his implosion limit and needed peace and quiet, but his mom was there pretty much chatting most of the time.

He told me he no longer could take having Claudia there, and he asked me to talk to her about going home early. On the one hand, she understood because she could see how stressed out Nick was. But on the other hand, she just did not understand why her style of expressing caring and intimacy was not compatible with what he needed at the time. Her feelings were hurt, but she changed her plane reservation and went home after a few days instead of staying the full week.

It took a long time for my scars to heal and to not feel aches and pains. The straw-sized hole where they pulled the duct out hurt more than the surgical incision because the skin had been growing really tight around it. It felt like it was ripping something out. I was walking around fairly well, although I did not have a lot of energy in the beginning. At first I would walk around the house, then Nick and I would walk around the cul-de-sac by our house, gradually extending the number of times we went around it.

It was a long time before I could lift anything of any substance and do anything and resume my quasi-normal schedule. The recovery time took much longer than I thought.

Dear Dear Leah,

I hardly know what to write, but I want you to know how much you matter and that I am thinking of you. It's strange to suddenly realize how much a person is integrated into your life; the books you loaned me sit on the stairs so I won't mix them with others, the cat vase you bought for me watches me from across the room, it's time for our birthday lunch.

Please call on me for whatever I can do—drive you to appointments, to cover Nick's classes so he can drive you, feed your dogs—whatever.

With love,
Virginia
[Card from friend and department colleague, Virginia)

Date: Fri, 10 Oct 2003
From: Peter
Subject: Your news
Dear Nick,

In the tumult of all that is to come, don't lose yourself in the fight. Take care of yourself. Be willing to ask yourself what that means to you, each day. You know that Susan and I will give you and Leah whatever support and respite you need. Just ask.
Peter

(Leah and Nick's friend, Peter)

When Leah came home from the hospital, many of our friends asked what they could to help, such as mow the lawn or wash dishes or make food for me. I rejected most of these offers, in part, because they wouldn't know where to put the dishes and I would have to tell them anyway. But I also appreciated doing everyday chores because they seemed to be therapeutic to some degree and they grounded me with at least some sense of normal reality. I remembered a scene from the movie "Oh God," when God—in the form of George Burns—first appears to John Denver in his bathroom. God tells John Denver to brush his teeth or shave because it will help him feel normal.

In retrospect, I wish I had accepted more offers from people to help, not for our sake, but for *their* sake. I learned that friends and family have a need to be involved more than simply saying prayers and having good thoughts. They wanted to feel as if they were doing something tangible for us.

When Leah began treatment, we started to let friends and family do more to help out. One student insisted on cleaning our toilets, although I refused to let her do it. Instead, she took Leah to a movie.

In contrast, a few friends and colleagues seemed to disappear completely. I ran into one of these friends at school and asked why she wasn't calling or visiting Leah. She said she knew Leah was dying and simply didn't know what to say, so she decided not to say anything.

Leah insisted that I continue to teach my classes. Fortunately, I only taught Tuesday and Thursday afternoon and night. If I had been employed in a 5-day-a-week job, I would have taken time off or shifted to a part-time basis.

I felt a lot of stress playing host to so many guests, but I knew Leah needed to see her family and close friends. After visits from Leah's dad and brother and then our friend, Laurie, my mom arrived. We had asked her to come because we thought Leah would need a lot of help, but she really didn't. What she needed the most was rest.

I was very behind in my grading and was still not getting much sleep at night. I hoped that with my mom there, I could catch up on my work and get some rest.

But my mom and Leah quickly resumed their usual pattern of talking and debating. I kept telling my mom that Leah needed rest, but every time Leah woke up she engaged my mom in conversation. I know Leah enjoyed their interaction, but it was driving me crazy.

The matter came to a head on the third night of my mom's visit. I had just taken a shower and was drying off in the back bedroom before dinner. I could hear my mom and Leah in some heated debate.

I went into the dining room and snapped.

"Don't you ever stop talking?" I said to my mom.

I don't remember what she said next, but it set me off.

"Why can't you just shut up?" I yelled.

"I knew this was going to happen," my mom said, after an awkward pause. "I knew you were going to break down."

I stormed out of the dining room, retreated to the back bedroom, and slammed the door. Leah came back and we talked. I told her that I needed my mother to go home. Leah agreed, and she asked my mom to leave the next day.

I dropped my mother off at the airport and went to my doctor and received a prescription for sleeping aids. That night I had my first full night of sleep in over 2 weeks.

I know that I didn't deal well with my mom's interactional style, and I am sorry for yelling at her and sending her home early. I was disappointed that she didn't understand my need for peace and quiet, and I'm sure she was disappointed that I didn't understand her need to interact with Leah the way they always interacted.

After my mom left, we didn't have any houseguests for a while. I took a sleeping pill each night for 2 weeks and recovered emotionally as Leah recovered physically.

Then we got ready for chemotherapy.

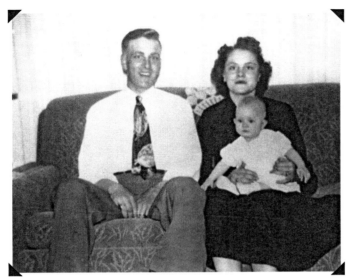

*Leah Rae
Vande Berg
with her
parents
Maurice and
Norma Vande
Berg, 1949*

*Nicholas Lee
Trujillo
with his
grandmother
Elsie Trujillo
Alcaraz,
1956*

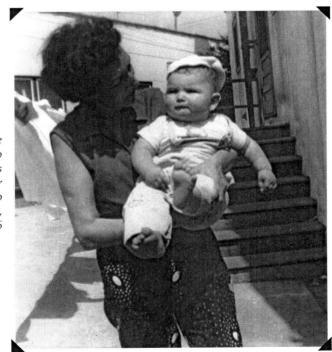

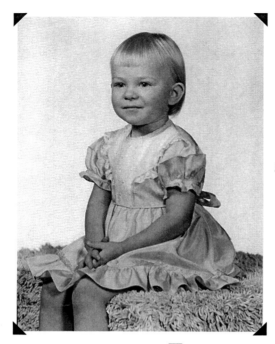

Leah Rae, circa 1952.

Nicky at his grandmother Marie Zwolinski's house, circa 1958.

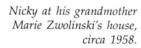

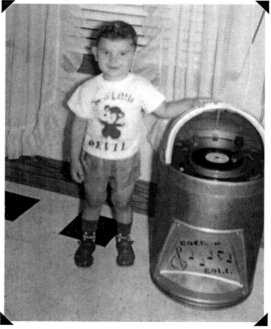

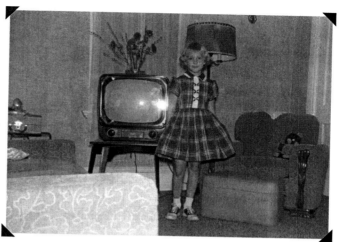

Leah, circa 1956.

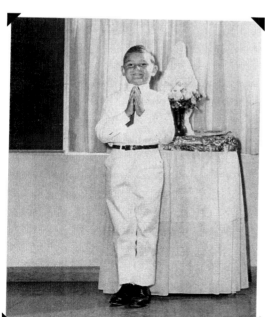

Nicky's First Holy Communion, 1962.

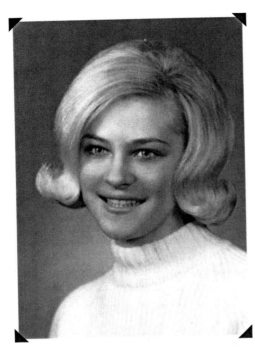

Leah's high school yearbook portrait, 1968.

Nicky's eighth grade class portrait, 1969.

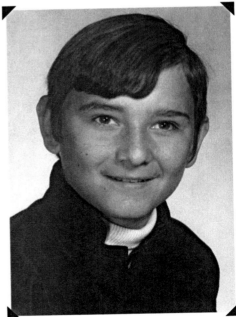

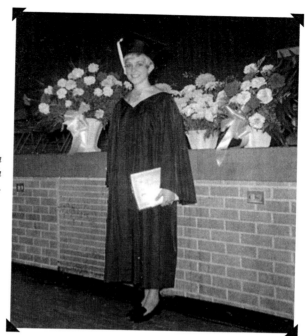

Leah's graduates from Sioux Center High School, 1968.

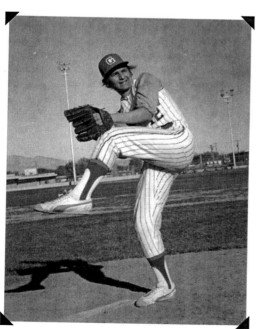

Nick pitches for Bishop Gorman Gaels, 1973.

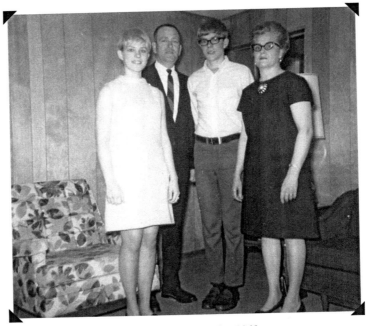

The Vande Berg family, 1969.

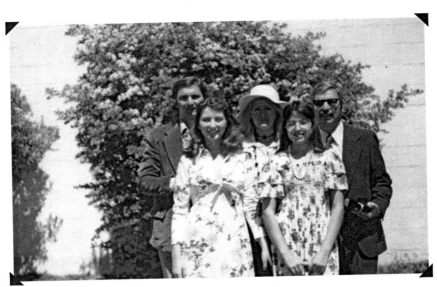

The Trujillo family, 1973.

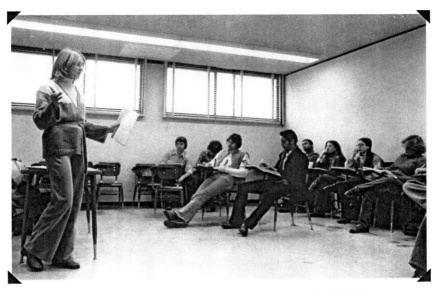

Teaching a class during her graduate program, circa 1979.

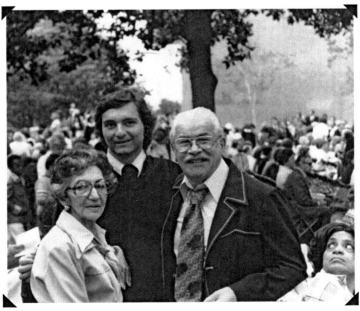

At Nick's college graduation, with grandparents Elsie and Pete Alcaraz, 1977.

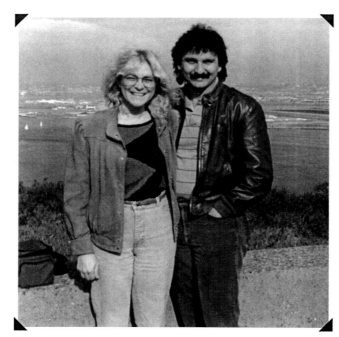

*In San Francisco,
on their
California trip,
1984.*

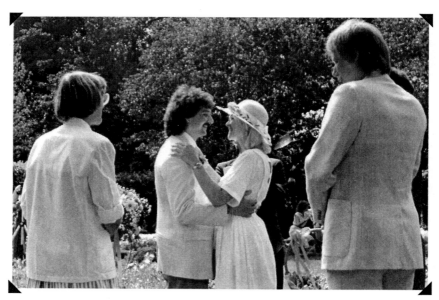

Their wedding, Evanston, IL, 1985.

At Sacramento State graduation ceremonies, circa 1995.

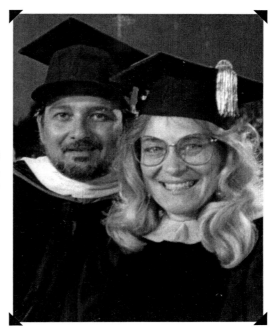

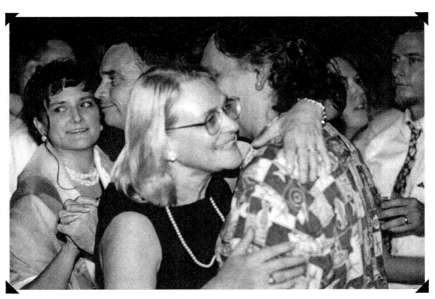

Dancing at a friend's wedding, circa 2000.

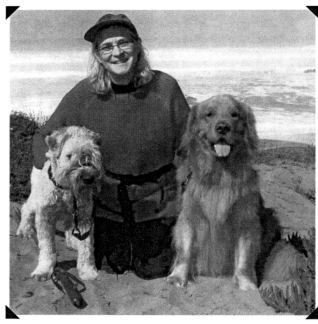

With Hawkeye and Ebbet in Fort Bragg, CA, the day after being diagnosed with cancer, October 2003.

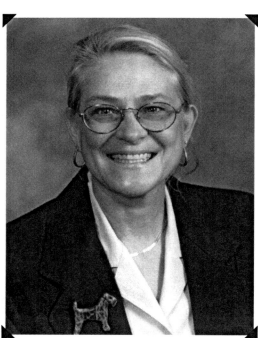

Leah, circa 2000, wearing her favorite pin, in the photo that was used for her funeral.

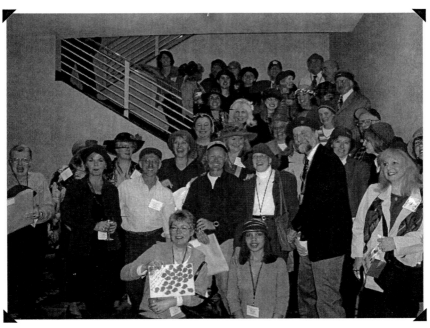

The "purple hat celebration" at the
Western States Communication Association convention, February 2004.

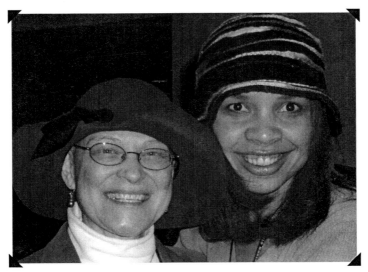

Leah with her graduate student "daughter" Jillian Tullis Owen, 2004.

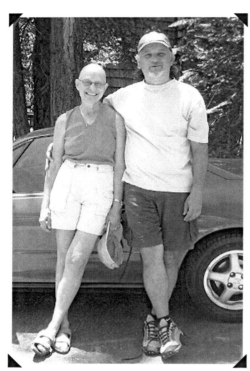

Leaning against Leah's "Little Red" car, Summer 2004.

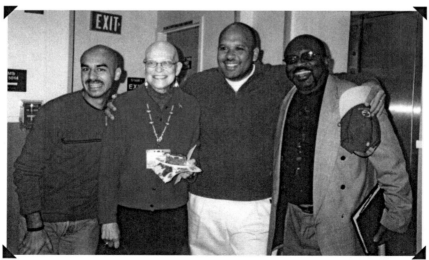

The bald heads of the Communication Studies Department: Diego Bonilla, Leah Vande Berg, Kimo Ah Yun, Donald Taylor, 2004.

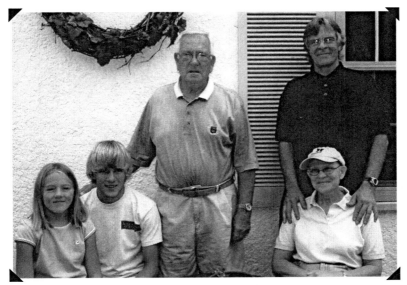

Leah with niece Anna Leah, nephew Austin,
father Morry, and brother Kevin, 2004.

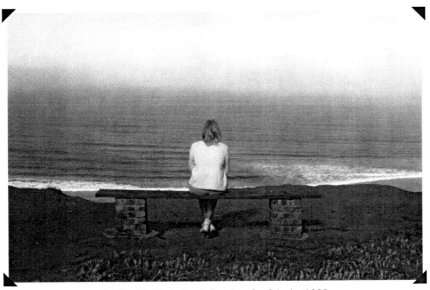

At the bluffs in La Selva Beach, CA, in 1990,
where some of her ashes would be scattered fifteen years later.

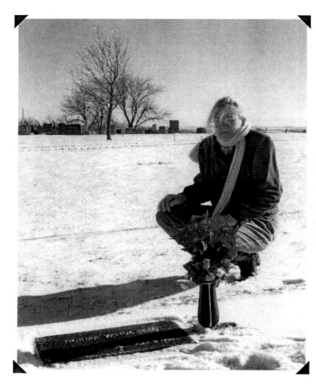

At her mother's grave in Sioux Center, IA, in 1990, where some of her ashes would be scattered sixteen years later.

Playing "Light My Fire" at Jim Morrison's grave in Paris, France, in 2007.

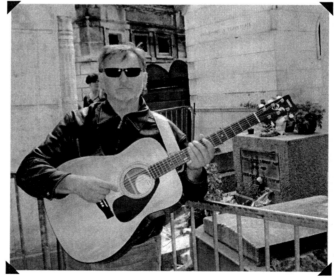

8

Chemo Reality

To: Leah Update List
From: nickt@csus.edu
Subject: Leah Update
Date: 11/16/03
Greetings — Leah and I had a nice day trip to the foothills today before she begins chemo tomorrow morning. She recovered well from her surgery and is ready to take on the next challenge, which will include 6-8 treatments of two kinds of chemo, 21 days apart....

   Thanks again for all of your gifts, cards, flowers, prayers, and good wishes. I'll keep you posted.

   Take care,
   Nick

A few weeks after my surgery, I met the hematology oncologist, a petite woman of Chinese descent. She seemed to be a little standoffish with me in the beginning. The first time she met with Nick and me about chemotherapy options, she mostly spoke to Nick and only glanced at me occasionally. When there were pauses in the conversation for answers, she would look at Nick, but I would answer. I found that exceedingly frustrating. I finally said to her, "You can speak to me." After that she was much better at looking me in the eye and talking to me. I think those are cultural differences, and they were a little challenging initially.

   She recommended, and we agreed, to do the most aggressive first-line treatment possible, which included three drugs: Taxol, Doxorubicin, and Sysplatin. Doxorubicin had a limited time frame in which it could be used because it is very hard on the heart.

The first day of chemotherapy seemed interminable. I was at the hospital from 9 a.m. to 5 p.m. They had to proceed very slowly with everything because they did not know whether I would have an allergic reaction to any of the drugs. They hooked me up to a machine and started the various intravenous drips of saline solution, antinausea medication, Benadryl, and then the chemo. The Bendryl immediately made me feel a little dizzy and groggy. The nurses wore plastic gloves and masks to administer the **Doxorubicin** because it is potentially toxic to anything it comes into contact with. It was a bright orange color.

The oncology nurses were wonderful, truly caring people with a calling and so warm and compassionate. They gave me hugs and had great eye contact and interpersonal skills. The oncology infusion suite actually is a pretty cheery place too. You sit in a reclining chair and they cover you with warm flannel sheets.

Throughout the day, I felt pretty liquid logged, although I got used to dragging my IVs with me to go to the bathroom. By the end of the day, I was really wasted. I was not yet nauseous, just exceedingly tired.

I went home and had a very light dinner of a few pieces of bland boiled chicken and vegetables. The next day, I awoke feeling positively rotten, as if I had been run over by a Mack truck and had the worst case of the flu I ever had in my life. My stomach was not entirely calm, and I felt like I could throw up at any minute if I thought about it. I also was a little bit light-headed. I took my antinausea drugs and spent most of that day and the next on the couch.

I was up walking around by Day 3, and I started to feel better by Day 4. By Day 5, I was feeling pretty close to normal and was able to go out and about and run errands to the grocery store. By Day 6, I could take the dogs on a 2-mile walk around our campus or along the American River.

That became my monthly regimen: 1 week of feeling rotten and 3 weeks of feeling good. I also needed to take injections to boost my white blood cells and shots to boost my red blood cells in-between, which Nick, bless his heart, gave me.

I initially was supposed to receive chemo infusions every 3 weeks, but after the second round it became clear that I was not going to be able to withstand treatments that often. We moved to once every 4 weeks, which my oncologist said was pretty typical. Very few people can stand the once-every-3-week treatments of all those drugs.

I realized how extraordinarily toxic chemotherapy was going to be to the healthy cells of my body as well as hopefully the cancer cells. I also knew how difficult it would be for my liver, which still had small growths that they were unable to remove during surgery. I knew that my liver was going to be working overtime trying to get rid of the cancer and still do its job, and that my kidneys were going to be flushing all of these toxins out of my system. From age 18 to 53^1/$_2$, I had done my fair share of drinking beer and wine, and in the summer gin and tonics. There also was a period where I drank fluffy little cocktails like tequila sunrises. I pretty much had the equivalent of a lifetime of enjoying alcohol, and so I decided that it was much better for my body to not drink anymore. I had entered my noncigarette-smoking phase 20 years before, and now I entered my nondrinking phase.

Once chemotherapy started, I lost the taste for alcohol anyway. The treatments changed how a variety of foods and drinks tasted. I completely lost my taste for wine. Even my favorite wines, like wonderfully silky smooth Chardonnays such as Ferrari-Cerrano, tasted like an old nickel. Red wine was a tiny bit better than white wine, but still it did not taste very good.

Instead of alcohol, I drank nonalcoholic ginger beer and ginger tea, which have an amazingly soothing effect on the stomach and on reducing nausea. My brother had suggested ginger, and I had no idea that it had such wonderfully positive antinausea properties.

I also started to eat marijuana brownies. Some of my friends with cancer had smoked pot, and it made all the difference in the world by helping them keep an appetite. I really did not want to smoke every day, and so one of my friends, who still is in many ways a hippie, although he is a professor and has raised a couple of kids, asked his wife to make me brownies with organically grown pot. The first batch was amazingly powerful. The brownies were an inch by an inch, and I cut them into quarters. However, the first time I took a full quarter, I became way too loaded and had to lie down for a few hours.

Although I was not at all hungry, the pot brownies gave me the munchies, and I was able to keep up my regular eating during chemotherapy. That is the reason residents of California approved the medical marijuana laws in the 1990s: to enable patients in my situation who are taking medication and feel nauseous to keep up eating and maintain their strength. Those pot brownies were a lifesaver.

The only time I ever threw up was when I was feeling so good on Day 4 that I did not take my antinausea meds. I threw up and continued to throw up for some time. After that experience, I learned that I needed to keep taking antinausea medication even if I did not feel nauseous.

In-between my chemo treatments, I was doing a variety of natural homeopathic treatments that my brother, a chiropractor and homeopathic proponent, had recommended. I read about them and I talked them over with my surgeon and my oncology doctor. Neither of them showed a lot of interest in alternative medicine. However, we agreed that I could take all of those alternative treatments as long as I stopped 2 days before my chemo and 3 days after my chemo so that any antioxidants that I was taking would not interfere with the chemotherapy.

I cut my hair very short before beginning chemo so it would not be such a huge shock when I lost my hair. After the third treatment, large clumps of hair started to fall out. Pretty soon I looked really scruffy, with tufts of hair here and bald spots there. One night I asked Nick to take his beard and moustache razor and shave the remaining hairs off my head, which he did, and I became bald. I thought I looked pale and emaciated without my hair. I looked like the people I see in photographs of prison camps from World War II.

I decided that I was not going to wear a wig. I have always worn hats as an adult anyway, and I have many of them. When it was too cold for me to go out without covering my head, I wore a hat.

I discovered that not every hat is warm and cozy. It makes a huge difference if the hat has a loose weave or not. If it is a loose weave, the wind can whistle right through it.

Whenever I was out in public, I felt that people were staring at me. We do not have a lot of bald women in our society, and people could tell that I was bald even if I was wearing a hat or a cap. Many people would smile, but then quickly look away because they were uncomfortable. Other people seemed to find me strange or scary, and they would look at me in strange or scary ways. I was not frightened, but it was clear that my appearance made quite a number of people uncomfortable. Over time I became used to that.

My family and close friends, however, teased me about my hair and acted like it was normal. They went out of their way to make me feel comfortable about being bald.

It was incredibly weird losing hair everywhere on my body. I lost nose hair, I lost the hair on my arms and legs, and my pubic hair. I felt like a newborn. Even when you shave you have a little stubble, but even that was gone. It was like I had baby skin. I used thick body lotion to make sure that my skin stayed soft and did not crack and get really gross, especially those places that had always been somewhat protected by hairs.

One night before Nick and I went to dinner, I started to put on new mascara, but I realized that I did not have any eyelashes or eyebrows. That was the first time I realized that my eye lashes had fallen out, and I really didn't need to put on mascara.

Nick and I went a long time without having sex. We could have had oral sex, but after my treatments my mouth was sore for at least a week and a half. Cancer puts a crimp in your sex life for a while, that is for sure. A long while.

Throughout my chemotherapy, I read a lot of sacred and meditative readings, including books by C. S. Lewis. Some of his writings are densely philosophical, and I am not a philosopher with a philosopher's mind. Many of his works, however, are quite accessible. One of my favorite books that include thumbnail versions of his arguments is called *God in the Dock*. In chapter 7 of that book, called "Scraps," he says praying for particular things always seemed to him to be advising God how to run the world. Lewis asks whether it would be wiser to assume that God knows best.

I never doubted for a minute that God would take care of me and give me the strength to deal with this, although I never dreamed that dealing with cancer would be one of the tests that he would ask me to face. I talked to God and told him that I did not understand why this was happening to me. Not that I am more special than anyone else, but I did not understand why this, and why now? What have I not done? What lessons had I not learned in the past that I now am supposed to learn from this experience?

One of the lessons God might have wanted me to learn is that I labor under the illusion that I am in control of the direction of my life and what is around me. In addition, I believe that this life on earth really is not the most important life. However, I have not lived my life this way. I have always been much more focused on the day after tomorrow rather than on the hereafter tomorrow.

I realize how extraordinarily privileged I have been in my lifetime, to be born in my family in this country at this time. I have been given so much, and I took so much for granted. I assumed that I would always have time enough to do all kinds of things, and I did not always put my spiritual life in the forefront of my life.

My cancer might have been a wake-up call to get my priorities straight and to focus on the important things. The important things are not getting these administrative reports done or working an extra session to replace the Berber carpet in the dining room. The most important thing is to quit thinking I can do everything myself and to trust God.

I do believe that if we believe, if we absolutely totally believe, that God can heal us, then God can intervene and heal us. I do believe that, although sometimes I wonder whether I believe in this enough.

```
To: nickt@csus.edu,  vandegerlr@csus.edu
From: Catherine
Subject: Assistance
Date: 10/19/03
```

Dear Nick and Leah,

Kimo and I would like to help make things easier for you. Consequently, we have come up with the following list of things we thought we could do to help. (I think it will be obvious which suggestions are Kimo's).

1. Walk and/or visit dogs while Nick is at the hospital.

2. Clean the house.

3. Yard care — mowing the lawn, watering, etc.

4. provide transportation to/from the airport for visiting family and friends.

5. Take "Little Red" out for a spin.

6. Let Nick win at golf.

7. Run errands/do grocery shopping.

And, of course, anything else that comes to mind.

You are both in our prayers.

Much love,

Catherine and Kimo

On her first day of chemotherapy, Leah expressed concern about catching a cold to one of the nurses.

"I wouldn't worry about the flu," the nurse said and laughed. "You have cancer!"

Welcome to the world of cancer jokes.

I worried that the chemo would really debilitate Leah, but after a few days of rest on the couch, she was fairly strong. She could even go on our normal walks along the river.

One of the hardest things I had to do during this time was to give her shots to keep up her red and white blood cell levels. I have always hated needles. I closed my eyes when I had blood tests and when Leah gave allergy shots to our Airedale terrier, Ragbrai. But Leah couldn't give herself the shots, so I had to learn how to do them. The first time I did it was challenging, but then I gave them to her with ease.

Leah remained very upbeat during chemotherapy. She maintained her trademark smile, and every day she said, "Have I told you how much I love you today?"

I tried to make a little time for myself as Leah got into a routine during her treatments. I had mostly given up golf and tennis, but I took long walks with the dogs during her couch time in Week 1. Doing something physical in nature cleared my head and helped me think about anything besides her cancer. The walking also helped me keep my weight down, as I was eating some of those organic brownies with her.

Leah was so strong and positive during her months of chemo that I felt I had to be strong too. But it wasn't always easy.

One night a couple days after her treatment, Leah and I sat on the couch holding hands. I was feeling very tired and beat down, and I told her I didn't think I could teach the next day and might call in sick.

"Would you like me to guest lecture for you tomorrow?" she asked and smiled softly.

"I guess I will be teaching tomorrow," I said and laughed. Leah desperately wanted to teach but couldn't do so, while I could but didn't want to. But I bucked up and did my job.

In some ways, dealing with Leah's cancer was incredibly hard, but in another sense, it wasn't. When something like this happens to you, you have no choice but to kick into another gear. Quite simply, you just find a way to do it.

Her cancer also made me stop whining about things like nagging aches and pains, car problems, office politics, and other aspects of daily life.

For example, during this time, my department had a chair that, in my opinion, was a bully who picked on part-time instructors and untenured faculty members. As a tenured full professor, I felt I needed to do what I could to protect my junior colleagues, so I butted heads with this chair on numerous occasions. We exchanged flaming e-mails, and I filed formal complaints against him to deans and school administrators.

But when your spouse gets cancer, even office bullies become less important. I stopped engaging in office politics with him and devoted all of my attention to my wife.

While Leah maintained her strong faith in God during her cancer, I have to admit that my spiritual life suffered a bit. I believe that if there is a God, he (or she) chooses *not* to intervene in human affairs. And so I did not find comfort when people of faith told me that Leah's cancer was part of "God's plan." I wondered why any God would want someone to suffer like that. During this time, I attended church with Leah every Sunday, and I found some comfort in ritualistically saying Catholic prayers, but I couldn't find any deeper meaning in her cancer. To be honest, I didn't really try to find such deeper meaning through prayer or church. But I am really thankful that Leah's faith gave her such strength.

I continued to send Leah updates through e-mail, although these updates evolved from earlier clinical descriptions of her condition to very personal disclosures about the emotions we felt as we went through this ordeal. Friends forwarded my messages to other friends, and soon there were over 200 people on the "Leah Update List." One day I received an e-mail from a colleague in another state asking me to "subscribe" her to the list. I replied that it wasn't a subscription, but I would add her name to the list of names I had created.

If I had been afflicted with cancer, I probably would have sent one e-mail to a select group of friends, telling them I had cancer and that I might disappear for a while. I'm pretty sure I would keep my feelings about it to myself.

At first, I found Nick's e-mails about Leah distasteful. They seemed too private to share with so many people in such a public way. I would be more private about this. But as time progressed, I changed my mind and found them a beautiful way to share the joys and sorrows of core life struggles, and I found Leah's energy in the group that shared her news. I feel that Leah lives more visibly to me through the stronger friendship ties she gave me as we shared her passage together.

(Our friend, Janellen)

```
To: Virginia
From: vandeberglr@csus.edu
Subject: Re: HOW ARE YOU?
Date: 12/6/03
```
Dear Virginia: I am good! I have felt really quite normal the past 2 weeks. I have learned from this round that Week 1 is awful for 4 days, but on Friday I begin to feel human again, and then I have 2 great weeks (with just a little tiredness at the beginning). So, yes, I definitely would like to go out for a cup of tea. That would be quite splendid!

I have chemo on Monday the 8th, so 8-11 are out. The 12th is possible, as are the 17th through

the 19th. Call (and talk a while because sometimes
I am in the other room and it takes me a while
to get to the telephone).

I am tentatively planning to go to graduation
because Anne says James is intending to walk. I
won't stand up and shake hands with all our grads
(too many germs for my immune system), but I will
shake hands with James and Alexis and whoever else
among the grads is walking. We also intend to
join the department Christmas party at Ray's for a
short time.

My current plan for next semester is to work
half time in administration (that gives me a
flexible schedule, so I can schedule meetings
for days I feel good). Teaching would necessitate
that I cancel my classes 1 week out of 3 — the
week after chemo when I lay on the couch, nauseous
and moaning all day — and I think that would
be too disruptive. I will serve on the grad
committee and supervise the COMS 5 TAs, too,
so I will be in the department at least
occasionally.

Hugs,
Leah

Cal and Susan, our friends from Fort Bragg, moved to Santa Barbara for the
winter that year, and they invited us to stay in their house in Fort Bragg
during our winter break. We accepted their offer and headed for the north
coast the day after Christmas. We spent about 12 days there before I had
to return to Sacramento for chemotherapy.

Two friends, Peter and Susan, joined us for 3 days from Washington.
We had the most splendid and delightful visit, just cooking and talking and
eating and walking. I remember a particularly entertaining conversation we
had one night about what kind of dog each of us were and Peter becoming
quite surprised when the three of us agreed that he was a little terrier.

After Peter and Susan left, Nick and I stayed there with the dogs. We
would sit at each end of their long harvest dining room table. To our right
or left, depending on which end of the table we were sitting at, was a mag-
nificent panoramic view of the ocean. We worked on various book projects,
prepared meals, took walks, and went into town to the bookstore.

We also took pictures of water tower houses because we had decided that we would build our guest cottage with that architectural design. We could not afford to build the main house until we retired, but we thought we could start building the cottage. Although we had been going up there for many years, we discovered to our surprise and amazement that there are a large number of water tower houses. Some of them were actual water towers that had rooms in them as part of hotels, but most were houses with a water tower design.

Cal and Susan had disconnected the satellite service and did not have a functional TV, so we did not fall into our usual habit of sitting on the couch after dinner and turning on the TV and desultorily watching whatever was on. Instead, we listened to the local radio station, KOZT, or "the coast" as locals call it. On New Year's Eve, the station played the top 95 songs of all time, as their frequency is 95.3 on the FM dial. Nick and I each made a list of what we thought would be in the Top 10. We listened to the countdown, and I drank a few sips of champagne after dinner. It was a delightfully relaxing nontelevisual New Year's Eve.

In February, Nick and I flew to our regional convention in Albuquerque. I had chemotherapy on a Thursday, and we flew to New Mexico on a Saturday. I really was not feeling very good yet, and I passed out on the plane briefly, which freaked out Nick and the flight attendants. However, I made it, and we had a great convention.

At that conference, my friends, unbeknown to me, organized a purple hat night at the big cocktail party on the first night. The association used to have a purple clothing day for women as a symbol to signify being feminist. All of my friends and colleagues and students came in moral support wearing purple hats. There were hundreds of purple hats. It was really quite extraordinary and so wonderfully heartwarmingly comforting. I had always felt that this association was like a family, but never so much as that night.

I had been elected vice president of this association, and I decided that I would continue to keep the position rather than resign. I thought that I would be able to get through the first round of chemotherapy when I was vice president elect, when there is not a lot of responsibility. I truly believed that I would be cancer-free by the time I became vice president and president.

I completed my 8-month regimen of chemotherapy in June, and a CT scan at that time showed that the tumors in my body had shrunk significantly, down to one very small growth on the side of my liver as well as another tiny one that seemed to be floating around. My oncology doctor said I needed to take a break from chemotherapy, for my body and for my heart, and that was fine because I felt great.

In July, 1 month after my last chemo, my hair started to grow back. I had hoped that it might grow in red and curly, but it grew out to about a half an inch of gray stubble.

In the summer, we went camping on the coast and to a wedding in southern California, and I went to Iowa and Indiana to visit my family and friends. Nick also was great about taking us on drives to places we had never been before. I have always found it very soothing to drive because it takes me out of my typical time–space continuum.

As the summer started to fade, I became very excited. Autumn is my favorite season. I love the smell of walnuts when they fall to the ground on top of the leaves and start molding a little bit. It is a wonderful rich kind of perfume. The colors are so rich and vibrant.

Fall also means going back to school, and I cannot think of anything I would rather do than teach, except maybe be the TV critic for *The New Yorker*. Nick had asked me what I wanted to do when the fall semester started, and I said I wanted to go back to full-time teaching.

There were some pragmatic reasons for my decision. Economically, for our lives not to fall apart, I could not simply quit teaching. We have a range of commitments, and I did not think I could just withdraw from them and radically change the quality of our remaining lives together.

However, the main reason that I continued to teach was because it helped me to continue living in the here and now. The scriptural readings and meditation I did helped to prepare me for dying, but I needed to continue to do what I loved to stay positive. Teaching is how I communicate what is important to me, what I believe, and what I think will help other people. If I were not going to die in a car accident, I would have time to reflect on the importance of living and dying and on how to live and how to die, and I could teach others about living and dying. Traveling or doing a mission would be great, but going in and teaching every day was my mission.

As the first day of the semester approached, I became very excited. I always used to get really nervous before the first day of classes, but I approached that semester rather differently and did not feel nervous. I made the decision that I should savor every day and be thankful for every day.

Around this time, I had an occasional upset stomach, but I assumed that my body was just getting tired of all of the iron and everything else I was still taking. I knew that I had another CT scan coming up in September, and I believed the results would be positive.

After Leah was released to go home, she insisted that Nick return to work. I was available on the days he taught and was happy to help. The first day I went over, she was sitting on the couch and eating solid food, and she was extremely optimistic about her recovery. We talked for a while and then I asked if there was anything that I could do: vacuum, wash dishes, laundry? She refused at first, but I managed to convince her that as one of five children in a large active family, I was used to doing chores.

I straightened the kitchen, swept the floor, vacuumed the carpet, and washed a few loads of laundry. Leah woke up after a nap and was happy to see what I had accomplished. She talked about her family and how far away they were and how she and Nick had always been self-sufficient. I told her that times like this were when she needed to let people help her.

"Focus on your body, your health and your relationships," I said. "Everything else will get taken care of."

From that day on, she allowed me to clean, make her meals, take the dogs for walks, change the sheets, and do laundry. I think it helped her to conserve her energy for fighting the cancer.

(Leah's former student, Juliane)

To: Leah Update List
From: nickt@csus.edu
Subject: Leah Update
Date: 1/14/04
Hello All —

Leah had her third chemo — five more to go — and is responding very well. The latest CT scan was 90% positive, according to the docs. It showed that all of the lesions identified previously have decreased significantly and the fluid identified previously has resolved. The only negative was that a previously unidentified small growth (2 cm) was found in the pelvis, which might have been hidden in fluids in previous scans or might indicate the presence of a new growth. But all in all, the docs say the scan was very good and shows that the chemotherapy is definitely working. Leah continues to handle the chemo very well. She has lost her hair — and over the holidays I shaved what was left of her comb-over — but she continues to experience only moderate nausea and fatigue for a few days after the treatments and then is her usual active self. Her blue eyes continue to sparkle.

We had a great holiday, spending 2 weeks in Fort Bragg, CA, at our friends' great house near the beach. Now we're getting ready to go back to school; Leah will be back part time doing administrative work and advising. For those in the field, Leah and I will be attending the WSCA conference in February in Albuquerque, so we hope to see some of you there.

Thanks again for all your support and prayers. Have a happy and healthy '04.

Take care,
Nick

The trip to Fort Bragg right after Christmas that year was definitely bittersweet. We talked with great excitement about building a guesthouse and even drew up some tentative plans, but I secretly felt she would not be around to see that guesthouse. I also recognized that she was in no condition to begin what usually is a pretty stressful process of building a house. But I maintained my enthusiasm around Leah, mostly to keep up hope.

The convention in February was wonderful. I'm not sure I have ever been as moved as when I saw what seemed like hundreds of people at the convention kickoff wearing purple hats. Before we arrived, Leah was wearing a brown or black hat and I suggested that she wear a purple one. She declined, saying it didn't match her outfit. I had been informed of the purple hat fest by Leah's friends a few days before the conference, and I told them I would get Leah to wear a purple hat.

"Leah," I said sternly. "Do not argue with me. Just trust me and wear a purple hat."

She complied and then experienced one of the most loving gestures of support her friends could have given her. I felt badly for the people without purple hats who did not get word of the gesture from Leah's friends, but they were very supportive.

Our sex life pretty much ended with her diagnosis. We were married for almost 20 years and she went through menopause, so we had gone without sex for weeks at a time. But after surgery, Leah was in pain and during chemo she was nauseous and weak, so I waited for her to take the lead.

Leah showed no interest in sex at all until after her last treatment, more than 8 months after her surgery. She asked the chemo nurses about it, and she told me they said she could have sex. It was a Saturday morning, and we got naked in bed.

But Leah couldn't quite get into a comfortable position, and I felt very uneasy when I saw her completely hairless. Some guys may have a fetish for hairless women, but I do not. It didn't even look like Leah. Neither one of us had an orgasm, and we did not try again.

As the summer faded and the beginning of the new semester approached, I asked Leah what she wanted to do about school. Without even taking a moment to think about options, she said she wanted to return to full-time teaching.

I lobbied for us to take a leave and travel to Holland and other places in the world. She countered that we would have our sabbatical leaves the following year and could travel then. I wasn't sure if she would be there then, although I didn't say that. She also argued that we couldn't afford to take a leave. I told her we had plenty of money in the bank, and I also knew that we had sizeable life insurance policies for both of us, although I didn't say that either.

As usual, Leah won the argument, and it was appropriate for her to win. When you have a terminal illness, you get to pick what to do with the rest of your life. I very much like teaching, but if I had been diagnosed with cancer, I would have quit my job and gone to Australia and spent my last months lying on the beach.

But I understood that teaching was Leah's passion, and if she were to give up that passion, she would be giving up hope as well. She was so overjoyed to get back in the classroom.

9

Back With a Vengeance

To: Barbara
From: vandeberglr@csus.edu
Date: 8/20/04

Thank you for the reply and confirmation. My summer turned out to be busy too, and like you, I have stayed away from school except for meeting with COMS 5 TAs. I am back (as of yesterday) after a visit to Indiana (my buddies at Purdue & Butler), Iowa (my father and his wife), and South Dakota (my brother and his family).

I am delighted to hear that your colonoscopy results were so good.

I am in limbo. A lesion remains on my liver. We don't know if it is scar tissue or cancer or a combination, and there is really no good way to find out (surgery to remove it would be very risky — I would lose six quarts of blood and the survival rate for that surgery is about 60/40; biopsy is not particularly useful — this is one of those times when sampling theory does not necessarily provide useful predictive results since the slices picked might be only scar tissue while the tissue slices next to them, which were not sampled, would be cancer, plus that would be another surgery).

So, I am taking a break from chemo, and in September considering a somewhat untried chemo that has been used with some other types of cancer but not ovarian/uterine. And having done some more research, I am asking my surgeon this week about possibly doing radiowave oblation of the remaining

```
lesion.  I  have  blood  tests  and  another  CT  scan  in
September  to  see  what  has  happened  since  June.
    Doing  nothing  and  waiting  is  a  bit  stressful,
though  I  feel  good  and  now  have  hair  fuzz  starting
to  grow.  Please  keep  me  in  your  prayers.
    Warmly,
    Leah
```

My first day of classes was truly a delight. I loved being back in the classroom, chatting with my colleagues, meeting with my students, doing everything that defines me as a professor. I was filled with so much joy and happiness. I remember saying, "Thank you good and gracious God for my life."

I knew that I had to go in for the CT scan in early September, and I was expecting good news. What I received, however, was a body blow. The cancer already had grown back. The lesion on the liver, which we did not know was cancerous or simply scar tissue, also had grown. I had spots on the wall of my abdomen. I had a mass growing between my kidney and my ureter.

I was really angry that the cancer had returned so quickly because I was so confident that I was going to be able to overcome this. However, it became quite clear to me that the chemotherapy was not working, and I was not getting better. I realized that I had gone through all those treatments, and yet I might not be able to finish my fall teaching or do my association responsibilities with the energy and verve that I expected. For the first time, I let myself feel sad and discouraged, rather than optimistic and hopeful, and I finally let out my pent-up emotions.

When the chemotherapy had worked so well, I truly believed that God was using modern medicine to help heal me. When I was not healed, I said, "Okay, Lord, what does this mean?" I knew that when I asked him to heal me, his answer very well could be, "Not in this life, Leah."

But I never doubted my faith. I do not know whether my cancer is part of God's plan. I do not know that natural evils like this are part of what God intends for the world. I do not think God intended that there would be evil in the first place. I consider cancer to be a natural evil. It is an evil related to our being biological entities who have manipulated our world in such a way that we have caused mutations and created this disease. For example, because of our desire to raise more and more corn on fewer and fewer acres, we use a variety of chemical fertilizers, which have negative effects on the land and the water and the products and the people who use them. In that sense, I think it is an evil of our own making.

I admit that I have not always necessarily listened to what God wanted me to do. One of the other things I prayed about when I got cancer was for God to let me know how he wanted me to spend the rest of the time I have left. When my cancer initially responded so well to the treatments, I thought that maybe God had some multiyear plans for my life. Then when I had the recurrence so quickly, I reacted with the propensity to think as a foolish little human being and believe that I could argue and negotiate with God. Oh, could I please have a little more time? When it came back so soon, it seemed to me that the answer was, "No, I don't have any further plans for you. I need for you to witness now where you are, to let me live and speak through you now and through what you are doing, and to learn what I need for you to learn right now."

However, I did not give up. I started a new type of chemotherapy because the treatments I had been getting did not work as well as we had thought. By the end of my 8 months of treatment, though, my veins were pretty brittle, and so I needed to have a port, an implant that goes directly into a vein underneath the skin on my chest. The surgery was very easy, and they do not even put you under a general anesthetic. It ached where they put the port in for a few weeks, but it took a longer while to get used to that little Borg-like implantation.

By the time October came, I realized that I was a 1-year survivor. However, my life at that time was not going very well. I had to have a blood transfusion because my red and white blood cell count was very low. My stomach and abdomen also were much harder and more distended, which meant that aceitis fluid was building up. I also needed to take natural laxatives to keep my bowel movements loose and regular because of a hernia that we discovered a couple of months earlier.

Then I had to have a stent put in. A tumor was surrounding my left ureter, and the doctors feared that it would block it and I would have liquid left up in my kidney not being able to drain to my bladder, which could cause an infection. They put a little tube in to help my kidneys drain like normal again. I will always remember the presurgery consultation with the doctor. She was wearing really fashionable spiked high heels, the first time I had ever seen a doctor in her office wearing shoes like that. But she was very nice, and, although I had to have a general anesthetic, the surgery was successful.

Nick suggested that we go to the Netherlands for my birthday at the end of the month. We had never been there, and Nick made contact with my cousins who lived there whom I had never met. Our friend, Laurie, who travels a lot for business, gave us miles so we could fly business class for free. We had so much fun planning the trip and talking about all the places that we would go and stay. That was great because it is hard to find things that you can look forward to when you are at this stage in the disease.

Unfortunately, my condition deteriorated, and about 1 week before we were supposed to go we had to cancel the trip. I was hugely disappointed, but there was no way that I could have gone abroad at that time. My stomach was so bloated that I felt 9 months pregnant and I could barely walk. The doctor also was concerned that I might have a "catastrophic event" on the plane or become seriously ill in Europe and have to spend time in a Dutch hospital, where they did not know the details of my case. It seemed like the right decision to make at the time.

On the day before my birthday, my stomach was so bloated that I thought I was going to burst. I felt like I was 9 months pregnant, and, boy, did I develop a new empathy for pregnant women. I called my surgeon's office and spoke to the nurse practitioner. She told me to come in and she would tap my stomach. I arrived at the office and went across the hallway to the OBGYN so one of the doctors there could do an ultrasound to find a pocket that was good to tap. I went back to the nurse practitioner's office and she sterilized a small needle and stuck it in me, then followed that with antiseptic and a much larger needle. The second needle felt like a little bee sting, but that was it. Before I knew it, they had drained 4 quarts of water weighing almost 10 pounds.

I was able to stand upright and walk out of their office. I could breathe comfortably, and I did not feel that all my organs were being compressed. It was such a wonderful sense of relief.

The nurses in oncology had recommended against getting my stomach tapped because you can get an infection from the needles entering the cavity and because it is an artificial not a systemic solution to the problem. They understood why I needed relief, but they said the fluid would come back faster if I had my stomach tapped, and then I would have to keep having this procedure done more and more frequently. The hematology nurses are really more into the big picture of remission at this point than they are into pain management.

On my birthday, I opened my presents from Nick in the morning. I also received a bunch of sweaters and hats and gloves as well as lots and lots of flowers from friends, relatives, students and colleagues. Our home looked like a florist shop. They were visually gorgeous, although after a while it actually started to smell a little musty.

Pastor Carol picked me up about noon and we went to Whole Foods for lunch. I had a little Sonoma chicken salad and part of a Dolmathe. We had a nice visit, and then she brought me home. That afternoon, my student, Juliane, came over with some more flowers, and she massaged my legs to move the water buildup to my lymph system, which helped hugely.

That evening I ate a small portion of this absolutely exquisite steak that Nick cooked for me. The doctor had suggested that I should beef up my protein. At about ten to eight, Nick took me to my church choir's practice session. My church choir always felt like a little community to me, like a family of people who are sharing an idea and singing with one voice. A wave of peacefulness and serenity always came over me whenever I sang with my church choir.

They sang one of my favorite songs, "In This Very Room," and it really did feel like Jesus was there in that room with us. Afterward they sang "Happy Birthday" and had a cake decorated that said "Happy Birthday Leah."

It was a lovely birthday.

I had felt so rotten the previous weekend that I thought my family should come and see me sooner, rather than later. After I was drained, however, I felt so much better, and it was clear that I was not going to die within the next week or two. There was all the crisis and stress that Nick had been coping with regarding whether we should or should not go to Holland and seeing me in so much pain. He needed time to recover, and so he told me that he could not cope with a visit from my entire family then and that he wanted them to come a few weeks later. He said that if they came now, he would have to go away for a little while.

I knew that it had been a really stressful few weeks for Nick, and having my brother, sister-in-law, their two kids, and my dad and stepmom here all at once would have been very stressful. If I lived around them it would be different because they could drop in for a half hour at a time, but they are a long distance away. Nick had been such a rock, so positive, and I did not want him to have to leave his house. However, I have a different relationship with my family than he does with his family, and I do not think that he quite understands the bond that my family and I share. They would walk through fire for me. Whatever I asked, they would make it happen. So I called and talked to them about the situation, and they rescheduled their trip. They were delighted that I felt better. I was sorry I did not get to see them then, but I knew I would see them a few weeks later.

Over the next couple of weeks, I became really surprised and discouraged with the rapidity with which my health deteriorated. There were a bunch of things I thought I was going to be able to get done that I will not be able to do, and it was frustrating. Death never seemed quite that imminent before, but it started to feel very imminent.

I was hoping that Nick and I could go to our national convention in mid-November so I could say goodbye to that whole group of friends, but I was too sick to go on that trip, too.

Although I was not well enough to fly, Nick and I continued to do little day trips with the boys. We went to Bodega Bay on a beautiful autumn day. We went through Napa and Sonoma valleys, and the grape vines were turning yellow and red. It was just gorgeous.

Leah's birthday fell on a day when Nick was teaching, and he asked if I would go by the house. I brought flowers and gifts and an assortment of small desserts that she and Nick could sample. I told her that whatever she needed, she was to ask me for and I would be happy to help. She asked me to rub her legs.

In response to the treatments that she was receiving, her body was producing fluids that collected in her legs. The only way to reduce the swelling was to massage the legs so that the lymph nodes could remove the fluid.

I did not tell her that it felt awkward at first to place my hands on her body. I sat at the end of the couch with her legs across my lap as I had many times before with my mother, sisters, and close female friends. But somehow this was different. She was my professor, my mentor, my teaching supervisor, and the chair of my committee. And she was sick. I started at her feet and squeezed as I moved my hands up over her ankle, rubbing and pushing the fluid up her legs from the bottom up. Then I moved up over the knee to her thigh and pushed the fluid higher to the hip and groin where it could be absorbed by the lymph nodes.

We talked about how she was feeling and about my progress in the program. She wanted to know how I was doing. On her birthday, while she was suffering from the effects of chemotherapy and an untrained masseuse, she wanted to know how I was doing. I rubbed her legs. It was the least I could do to help.

(Leah's former graduate student, Juliane)

My last trip to see Leah was around her birthday. I remember being very sad to see how she had declined. Leah's face was pale, gray shadows consumed it. She was hugely swollen from the disease and very uncomfortable. She was having trouble eating anything but a few sips of soup. She looked scared to me and was,

I thought, short and a bit angry at everyone. She was, however, planning on leaving that weekend for the trip to Holland.

The next morning, Nick expressed some doubts about Leah's ability to go to Europe. I told him pretty directly that I thought it was crazy to consider. She was physically miserable, weak, and not able to eat but a mouthful or two. I felt bad for being blunt, but I thought Leah was much more ill than I perceived Nick did. We both wanted her to take the trip, nothing would have made me happier than to be able to send her.

The next morning, the three of us cried at the dining room table regarding the trip to Europe. At first Leah blamed Nick and me for not letting her go; she thought and said we were cruel. It was very painful, and it brings tears as I remember it. We reassured her that we wanted her to go, and the decision was hers to make. In the end, she decided not to go. It was incredibly hard for her to give up that dream because it meant the disease had won.

The clock over the mantle ticked away, and soon it was time for me to leave for the airport. Leah and Nick walked me out and hugged me goodbye like they had done dozens of times before. I could not let myself think this was the last time I would see Leah; nevertheless, I cried all the way to the airport.

(Leah and Nick's friend, Laurie)

When the semester started, Leah was beaming. She was back at work and couldn't be happier. I was very glad that she didn't listen to my arguments about taking a leave.

I know Leah was very optimistic about her CT scan. I was not as hopeful, but because the doctor said the cancer would not return for at least 6 months, I was not pessimistic.

Leah woke me up early in the morning the day her oncologist called with the results. Leah seemed upset, even angry, and I thought I had done something wrong, like maybe I didn't lock the front door or I left milk out overnight. Then she told me that her cancer had returned.

She left the bedroom, and I started to cry. But I quickly regained my composure and rushed out of bed to be with her. We held each other in the kitchen for what seemed to be a year. I am not normally a big hugger and usually squirm away after a few seconds. But this hug was different. Neither one of us wanted to withdraw, not knowing how many more hugs we would be able to share together.

When we finally let go of each other after several minutes, she kneeled down and hugged Hawkeye.

"I hope whomever you meet next is a dog person," she told me. Then she started to sob.

Predictably, she quickly regained her composure and turned to some student papers and an administrative report. I mostly sat in silence and stared. I felt as if I had been kicked in the gut or the groin. I knew a recurrence this quickly meant that she didn't have much time left.

I asked Leah whether she wanted to take a drive, but she said she had to finish up her work. I needed to get some fresh air, and I told Leah I was going to go for a short walk with the dogs.

The boys and I went to the usual spot on the trail by the river. I had mostly avoided thinking about Leah's death since her diagnosis and surgery, especially when the chemo worked so well and I thought she would live at least another year or two. But that morning, I couldn't shake the feeling that she might only have months or even weeks to live. So many thoughts filled my head. I wondered whether she would hang on until she was paralyzed and debilitated, barely conscious, maybe for several months. We had both decided that if we were ever comatose, we'd want life support cut off. That had always been a future issue, a conceptual matter, but now it felt like a reality. I couldn't bear the thought of her barely clinging to life for a long time, but I suspected that her cancer was too aggressive for that to happen.

I also started thinking about my life after Leah. I didn't want to think about it, but I couldn't seem to not think about it. Our plan had been to continue working until we built our house and retired on the coast, but I started to wonder if I would even build a house on our land or sell the lot and move somewhere else, like Big Sur.

For the first time I also thought about being a widower at age 48 or 49. I was so comfortable with Leah after nearly 20 years of marriage. I liked sitting on the couch reading together or rubbing her feet while she lightly tickled my forearm. But our marriage was about to end in the most brutal way. And then I would have to start dating again? The thought of dating and falling in love and getting married again gave me a chill. My second marriage was supposed to be my last one. The third time is not the charm.

I tried to shake these thoughts from my head, feeling guilty that I was even having them just an hour or two after Leah received the news of the recurrence. Then I came across a hobbled homeless woman on the trail. I realized that Leah had a horrible disease, but she was getting very good treatment, we lived in a modest but comfortable house, and we had two well-groomed dogs, great jobs, and very good lives. And I would continue to have my dogs, my job, and my home after Leah's death. This poor woman lived outside, pulled a cart with all of her earthly possessions, most of which she picked from the trash. I felt sorry for the poor woman, but I also couldn't help feeling sorry for Leah and for me.

When I returned home, Leah was crying on the couch. I rushed over and we cried together in each other's arms. She cried more that day than during the entire previous year.

We met with her oncologist that afternoon, and Leah decided to try new chemotherapy treatments. She would have to get a port implanted in her chest, and even though it was a routine surgery, it was yet another setback.

At the end of September, we needed to complete proposals for our sabbaticals, which would begin the following year if approved. It was difficult to think of proposing a new project for what seemed like an eternity away, but we knew we had to do it. I think for Leah it was a way of keeping hope, that next year we would be on leave together. For me it was a way of getting a semester or a year off to cope with what now would be a certain loss.

I couldn't think of anything to propose, and then I thought about writing a book about Leah's cancer with her. But when I raised the idea, she dismissed it quickly. She said she wanted to keep her work separate from her illness, and that made sense to me. But a few days later, she changed her mind, saying that she thought a book would be a good way to teach people about how to deal with cancer and with death. From that point on, we started to dictate our thoughts into a tape recorder, and we shared our vision of a possible book.

We submitted our sabbatical proposals by the deadline. I made a special request that university officials consider giving us an early sabbatical because we did not know whether Leah would be alive the following year. I didn't expect them to grant our request, as it would set a precedent they might not want to set, but I never even received the courtesy of a reply. All we received was the form letter indicating our sabbatical proposals had been received and were being processed.

Leah continued to teach for the next several weeks. Her new chemotherapy regimen was not as debilitating, so she only needed substitute teachers for the days when she received treatments. But as her health deteriorated, I knew she would have to quit her job at some point, and I knew that would be devastating for her.

Even as her conditioned worsened, Leah didn't lose her sense of humor. On one chemo day, she received a prescription from the oncologist for new meds. She held the prescription in her hand and seemed confused, not knowing where to put it. She grabbed her wallet, which was stuffed with assorted papers.

"You'll lose it if you put it there," I said.

"I will not," she countered.

"Yeah, famous last words," I said without thinking.

"Well, if those are my last words, you can put them in the book," she said and smiled.

"Good comeback," the nurse said and laughed.

October arrived, and on the 9th Leah became a one-year survivor, although we didn't feel like celebrating. But I knew her birthday was coming at the end of the month, and I thought we should do something really special.

I proposed to Leah that we go to Holland, a place we had never been. I offered to track down some of her distant relatives there so she could meet them. I was stunned when, without debate, she approved the idea.

We became very excited as we planned the trip. I talked to Leah's father to get leads on possible relatives, and I tracked down a distant cousin who lived in Amsterdam with his wife and child who agreed to show us around. Our friend, Laurie, gave us frequent flyer miles so we could fly business class. Leah and I created an itinerary together, and I made reservations for hotels and a rental car so we could explore the countryside after visiting Amsterdam.

Unfortunately, Leah's health continued to deteriorate. Her abdomen continued to fill with fluid until she could barely walk. I started to think that she might not be well enough to travel.

Laurie flew in for a brief visit the weekend before Leah and I were scheduled to depart for Europe. She was shocked at how badly Leah's health had deteriorated, and when Leah went to the bathroom, she told me it was not a good idea for Leah to take an international flight. Although I resisted at first, I agreed.

Laurie and I decided to confront Leah about the wisdom of the trip. Leah was very upset with us for not supporting her desire to travel. She had heard the same advice from the oncology nurses and the doctor who was substituting for her oncologist. But she ultimately realized she could not travel in her condition.

Leah's stomach continued to swell, and the day after we were supposed to be on a plane, the nurse from her surgeon's office advised her to have fluid drained. The chemo nurses had advised against that, but Leah decided to get her stomach tapped. She felt immediate relief, and we wondered whether she would have been able to go to Holland if she had been drained a few days earlier.

The next day, when we should have been in Amsterdam, we took the boys to the Sonoma Coast in the van. Near the tiny town of Two Rock Valley, we stopped at the "Little Amsterdam House of Oysters." Not exactly the Amsterdam we were hoping for, but we had a nice day on the coast.

Before she was drained, Leah had asked her father and step-mother and her brother and his family to visit because she was not sure whether she would last much longer. But after she was drained, she felt much better and didn't feel as if she would die anytime soon. I asked her to ask her family to postpone their trip for a few weeks. Laurie had just visited, as had a former student, and with the stress of the semester and the decision about Holland, I needed a break before having more people descend on the house. I also suspected that her family would not be able to afford to come in October and then again for Christmas, so I suggested to Leah that they come a few weeks later for an early Christmas. She was disappointed, but concurred with the decision.

In early November, the director of our university's choral group came up with the idea to surprise Leah with a group of people singing Christmas carols. He contacted many members of other choirs in which Leah sang, and I told most of Leah's friends and colleagues.

We set a date, and I contacted all the neighbors to let them know that many people might be descending on our little cul de sac that night. It rained all day long, but stopped about a half hour before visitors were supposed to arrive. I asked Leah to come outside to see some new Christmas lights I had put up in the yard. She resisted at first, but when I insisted, she finally agreed. I helped her to the door and flashed the outside light on and off, the cue for the group to start singing.

About 100 people started singing carols. Leah's face lit up, and I helped her to a chair I had placed in the driveway. They sang songs for about a half hour, and then one by one said goodbye to Leah.

The skies cleared and over 100 people brought the gift of song to your home in a magical way that moved all of us deeply. It worked out perfectly, and I was sooooo happy that everything fell into place. I could see Leah's face beaming in the dark, and I believe she was transformed with the mystery of it all. We certainly were. . . .

Thanks to all who became part of our human chain, and it was our privilege to spend that night on Bruhn Court.

God bless you both.

(Leah's friend and choral director, Don)

To: Sheryl
From: vandeberglr@csus.edu
Subject: GE Fall Newsletter
Date: 10/20/04

Friday is good. Maybe late morning — around 11 or so? Thursday is chemo and blood transfusions....

My friend, Laurie, from Alaska will be here so you will get to meet her, which will be nice. I am afraid that I just am not going to be able to finish out the semester. Unless the new chemo that I start tomorrow REALLY works, continuing to teach is just not going to be an option much longer. And that really makes me sad because I really did want to finish teaching one more semester. Ah well — lessons, lessons, lessons.

As the weeks passed and my disease progressed further, I continued to tie up various loose ends. I arranged for colleagues to take over my classes, and I informed the chair of the department that I would begin taking sick leave soon.

In November, a slew of guests came to say goodbye because we were not sure whether I would be here for Christmas. My friend, Candy, came to visit from Indiana. We talked about all of the times we had been there for each other: during graduate school with its challenges, during my divorce, and during her move to Purdue. We had some good hugs and some cries.

Nick, Candy, and I went up to the foothills to a Christmas tree farm and Nick chopped down a tree. Nick put up the tree and decorated it, and Candy put out all my Dickens Village decorations. So the house was set for Christmas, in early November.

Then my dad and stepmother came to visit. I think my dad was blown away at how ill I had become. He did not know how much my condition had deteriorated since he visited in the summer. We had a very nice visit. We went to Apple Hill near Placerville and bought some apples. Nick made fires, and we sat around in the living room and talked. I know it was hard for my dad, even though he is a strong man with great faith.

My brother, Kevin, sister-in-law, Deb, niece, Anna, and nephew, Austin, came shortly thereafter. Anna, Debbie, and I made pecan tassies, using the recipe my mom made on the first Friday in December every year. They were my favorite treats. Anna learned how to make them, and I felt I had passed on that little family tradition.

Then on Saturday night, Nick, by himself, made a complete Christmas dinner: turkey and stuffing and cranberries and green beans and mashed potatoes. It was truly delicious. I made the mistake of having cranberries, though, which had a little bit of horseradish, and stuffing, which had a little bit of green onions. I was fine until about 3 a.m. I had tried not to throw up for a couple hours, but then I just had to and was very miserable. Throwing up is never fun.

On Sunday morning, I still was not feeling well. The gang packed up their stuff and got ready to go. When they left for the airport, it was very sad. My brother kept thinking that a miracle still could happen, and, of course, miracles can happen. As I looked at myself realistically, however, what I saw was a rapidly deteriorating body and a mind that had some good days, but not so many anymore.

Nick's mom, Claudia, arrived the same day my family felt. Claudia had come to say goodbye, but also to attend a special showing of "The Vagina Monologues" that my graduate students had organized as a fundraiser for a graduate student scholarship in my honor. One of my former graduate students had flown in for Thanksgiving to see her mother, and she attended the show as well. She was not handling my dying very well, and she kind of lost it when she saw me. She also had a cold, so she could not come close and hug me because I was so susceptible to germs.

I was not well enough to attend the performance, but I attended a lovely reception beforehand that my graduate students had organized. I had a chance to talk to a lot of folks who came, including many of my female colleagues. There were probably 40 people there. It was just lovely.

A funny thing happened as we approached the theatre. There was an ambulance and a couple of paramedics outside of the theatre. Nick and I had the same reaction when we saw it: Oh, no, people are going to think that Leah has keeled over. But, in fact, a woman had collapsed during an earlier performance.

It was good to see the many people who visited us, but it was a little surreal because they all came to say goodbye to me. I will not get to see them again. It made me feel like I was just floating along.

We had been having conversations every week with my oncology doctor about whether we should cancel the treatments. In late November, we did a test for my heart function and it had dropped from 65% to 40% as a result of the new chemotherapy. The new treatment may have slowed the cancer down the previous 2 months, but it really did not seem to be working or improving the quality of my life. I really did not see any good reason to continue the treatments, and there did not seem to be any benefits from trying another new treatment. In consultation with the doctor and with Nick, I decided to stop all treatments.

After I made the decision, Nick and I went to say goodbye to the oncology nurses in the infusion suite. One of the patients there had just had an allergic reaction to a treatment, so all of the nurses were busy. But we waited, and then Nick went inside to see whether the nurses who worked with me the most were available to say goodbye. Two of them did. I was able to say goodbye to them and thank them for the really caring and professional treatment they gave me. Their jobs are brutally difficult to do, and yet they do it with joy and such a delightful sense of humor and compassion.

After I stopped treatment, the hardest thing was staying positive. I stopped throwing myself 100% into doing things in the here and now because I knew that I would not be here to finish them. I have always known that life is finite, but most of us act as if it is infinite or at least that death is some time decades and decades away. I humorously and sometimes judgmentally talk about my students who think that they are immortal and nothing is going to happen to them, but in many ways I have been the same. At an intellectual level, I have always understood that from the minute you are born and are growing, you are also dying. But from an emotional sense, I have not really thought about how precious every single day is and how best to use every day as preparation for another life. I have used almost every day as a way to accomplish things in this life by and large. Having cancer and having my faith has made me focus on the mortality, not the immortality that we typically feel about our lives. We do not know for certain whether there are years to come, and we should live every day with love and joy and exuberance and gratitude that we have this day and this place. I now understand that learning a new way of thinking about living, which involves living and dying, is painful and hard.

On the one hand, I want to get up in the morning and say hello and have a happy and cheerful day in my encounters with Nick and other people. On the other hand, I think, well, I do not have very many days left and how do I want to spend my precious few hours that I have today? We spend most of our lives mentally in the future, not in the present. We do things in the present, but think about what we are going to do after this. What is next is always what we are thinking. It is exceedingly difficult to think about there being no next here, at least here. I love Nick, the dogs, my family, and my friends, and I am very sad that I will not get to share the rest of their lives. I am sad that I will not get to see my niece and nephew graduate from high school and college and watch them grow up. It is clear that my life is coming to a close and the future is collapsing into the present. And that is very sad for me.

I also am a little angry. I always like to think that if I do everything right, I am in control and everything will come out fine. However, it is very clear to me that I am not in control of this disease, and I am not in control of how effective or ineffective treatments have been. I am angry that our country has not done enough research on reproductive cancers—not just on treatment, but also on early detection. I am angry because I had really hoped that this regimen would work, that medicine would answer my request for healing. But the answer I received was not yes.

I did not get angry with God, however. I prayed all the time, as do many people, but for whatever reason, God has chosen not to intervene in this illness. I did find the lectionary readings I had done reassuring, however, because they reminded me that, although I may not be able to understand the whys, I am not alone and God will be with me.

One of the readings I did during this period was scripture about the rich young ruler who asked Jesus what he had to do to gain eternal life in heaven. The scripture says that Jesus looked at him and said, "Sell all that you have and follow me." The rich young man turned away sadly, and Jesus told his disciples how hard it is for the rich to enter heaven. I read some of C. S. Lewis and other people's thinking about that passage, and, like them, I do not read the meaning of that story to be about money, but rather about giving up what is most important to you on this earth and loving Jesus and God more than anything else. I believe that is really the essence of the story of Abraham when God asked him to sacrifice his son, Isaac. He trusted God and was willing to do that and give up what he loved and valued most.

I was thinking about that story in terms of my cancer. To me the question is, am I willing to give up my life? Is that what I value most? That was one of the meditations about what I am reading and learning. I have to be willing to give it up, but that does not necessarily mean that God is going to require me to do that. Like in the case of Abraham and Isaac, God intervened. He said you have to be willing to do it, but I may not require it.

One possible answer to why I have cancer is that I love my life here so much. I love Nick and the dogs, my family, teaching and writing, and what I do. Any objective look at the amount of time I have spent on things would indicate that I value these earthly things far more than I value my religious growth and experience. Thus, one possible explanation of why I have cancer is that I have to take a larger eternal perspective and spend as much time on that part of my life as I do on the present part of my life. That is one of the things I have been thinking about as I struggle to understand why and what I am supposed to be doing now as I bear witness to my faith. Maybe it is to invite others to think about God and faith. I believe that is what we are supposed to do throughout our lives, but it is not such an easy thing to do.

To: vandeberglr@csus.edu
From: Vande Bergs
Subject: thanks
Date: 11/24/04
Dear Aunt Leah and Uncle Nick,

Thanks so much for having us to your house. It was good to see you again. I really liked making pecan tassies with you.

The dogs enjoyed their toys very much. Biscuit was playing with them when we got home from the plane trip. I hope you have a wonderful Thanksgiving in California!

Love,
Anna Leah Vande Berg

I remember holding Leah's hand the last time I saw her. We hesitated to talk about her illness. I think she was trying to protect me. I was so impressed with how well she handled it.

She was fighting to the end. That's what I'll remember about her.

Her whole life was cut off at the top of her career. It's still a mystery to me.

(Leah's father, Morry)

A flood of visitors came in the weeks to follow: first Leah's dad and stepmom, then Leah's friend, Candy, then a former student, then my mother, then her brother and his family. Everyone put on a good face, but it was so sad to watch them say goodbye to Leah for the last time.

The wife of a close friend of mine in the field came up with the idea to put together a big scrapbook for Leah with photos and messages from Leah's friends and relatives across the country. Dozens of people sent items to Sandra, and the book arrived by Federal Express in November. Leah loved it. I did too, although it seemed to be another way that people were saying goodbye to her.

Leah's health continued to deteriorate, and it was clear that the new chemotherapy was not working. We met with the oncologist, and Leah decided to stop treatments because they were not improving the quality of her life.

Before we left the hospital that day, we stopped by the chemo infusion suite to say goodbye to the nurses. A patient had just suffered an allergic reaction to a drug, so things were hectic. But two of the nurses who worked most closely with Leah were able to come out for a couple minutes. They hugged Leah, and I could see their eyes getting moist with tears. I don't know how these nurses are able to continue to do their jobs for so long, when most of the people they treat die.

In early December, I arranged for colleagues to take over my classes. And I waited for Leah to die.

10

Uv Üï

To: Leah Update List
From: nickt@csus.edu
Subject: Leah Update
Date: 12/8/04

    Leah is barely hanging on. She went to bed at 8 p.m. on Sunday night and didn't wake up until 2 p.m. on Monday. She had a bit to eat and then slept the rest of the day and into the night. Yesterday she slept for the entire day and did not eat, just drank a little juice. The hospice people said it could be very soon. They come again today at 1 p.m.

    She is not feeling any pain, just mild discomfort when she wakes up. She is in and out of consciousness throughout the day and night. I whispered in her ear that the boys (the dogs) and I will be fine, that everything is all right, and that it is okay for her to go. I cancelled my last week of school this week to be with her (colleagues have taken over for me).

    The wind has been blowing fiercely for the last few days during an intense winter storm. Knowing Leah, it sounds like there is a heated debate going on at the gates of heaven. I think it will be peaceful very soon.

    Nick

It is so hard to leave the people whom I love so much, especially Nick and the boys. Yet every day I wake up and ask myself, what am I still doing here? I get up and feel good for about an hour, and then I go lie down on the couch and sleep my life away. Right now I am having a hard time swallowing. It takes longer and longer for me to do simple things. I get tired walking from the bedroom to the bathroom. If I am just going to be a vegetable on the couch, I might as well be a vegetable on the couch for a short time.

Nick and I had a fight this week. Not unpredictable, I suppose. But this is part of loving through cancer, too. The argument was about my unwillingness to recognize my situation. I am trying to realize how frail and fragile I am becoming, how very little I actually can do, and how dangerous it is for me to do many things. Nick expressed concern that I walked over to my roll-top desk and stepped over a wooden box to get some papers. That would not normally seem like a particularly onerous or dangerous thing, but given the hospice nurse's discussion of the dangers during this phase, it was very timely. She talked about how the biggest danger that I face right now is not recognizing all of the places where I could fall down and be hurt and have no way of helping myself. Of course I pooh-poohed it.

Nick reminded me that it was the second time in 2 days that I had put myself in danger. Yesterday after dinner, I was trying to carry a smorgasbord of six different kinds of dressings back to the kitchen on a tray in my shaky and fragile condition.

That is the crux of the problem: my unwillingness to recognize that I am dying and that I cannot do everything I want to do. I have to say I cannot do some things and ask Nick to do them for me. He said he would no longer be able to trust me not to do something stupid, like step over boxes with sharp edges. He needs for me to acknowledge that I am dying. I do not seem to be facing this reality terribly well.

In the bed she will die in, my good friend's body contorted, limbs limp and intertwined, cheeks sunken as if puckering like we did when sharing a brew, me vowing to plant my own vines, crush my own grapes, make my own wine, we laughed thinking of the purple feet I'd have, but not caring. I hold her hand this last time, gently because she bruises easily, the color of wine.

winter sky
the contrail stretches
horizon to horizon

("Horizons," from a book
of haibun by our friend, Bill)

I was certain that Leah would die the night of Sunday, December 5th. As was typical of previous nights, she took a gasping breath once every 20 or so seconds and experienced brief convulsive tremors with her hands and body every 20 or so minutes. But that night she lay in bed calmly. When she finally fell asleep, she reached for someone or something with her arms. She also seemed to talk to someone, although I couldn't understand what she was mouthing.

During research for a book I wrote about my grandmother's life and death, I read about people with near-death experiences who say their spirits floated above their bodies and that deceased family members served as escorts to guide them. As Leah reached up, I looked around the room, searching for God, an angel, the spirit of Leah's mother, a beam of light, for any sign that she was being called.

"Do you see your Mom?" I whispered in Leah's ear. "Do you see God?"

Leah didn't respond.

At one point when I thought she was about to die, I gazed at the ceiling and actually waved.

"Goodbye, Miss Leah," I said. "Can you see us down here?"

Again, no response.

I stayed awake for most of the night watching Leah. I held her hand and whispered to her that the boys and I would be okay and that it was time for her to go.

I fell asleep around 4:00 a.m. and woke up a few hours later surprised that Leah was still breathing. I got up and fed the dogs and let them outside. I also telephoned the office receptionist and said I was calling in sick for the week—the last week of the semester—and I had arranged for colleagues to take over.

For the next 2 days, Leah did not get out of bed except to go to the bathroom, although she only peed twice each day and hadn't had a bowel movement for almost a week. She no longer reached up with her arms or talked while she slept. When she woke up for a few minutes every 5 or 6 hours, I offered her food and liquids. She ate a few crumbs one day, but otherwise just drank sips of orange juice.

During those 2 days, a winter storm hit northern California with fierce winds that knocked down part of our fence in the backyard. The following week, I would joke with Leah's Pastor that God had indeed called Leah on Sunday, debated with her at the gates of heaven, and then told her that HE needed a few more days to prepare for her.

The winds let up on Wednesday morning. Leah slept the entire morning and then, to my amazement, she got out of bed and walked into the living room. She ate a small salad and nearly tripped as she carried a tray of dressings.

I told her that hospice officials were coming to the house that afternoon. Despite my objections, she insisted on taking a shower before they arrived.

I placed the shower chair in the tub and helped her undress. I had seen Leah without her top whenever I placed a new pain patch on her back, and without her bottoms every night when I helped her change into her pajamas. But I hadn't seen her completely naked for several weeks.

I nearly collapsed at the sight. Her arms and legs were rail-thin, her entire ribcage protruded, and her stomach was severely bloated. She looked like a starving woman in a picture from the Holocaust or from a plague-ridden country in Africa. I maintained my composure, barely, and helped her wash herself and get dressed.

At 1 p.m., hospice officials arrived to finish processing Leah's case. Leah stayed awake for the 2-hour meeting as the nurse and social worker went over details, ranging from her various medications to the funeral arrangements. The nurse emphasized the risk of falling, although Leah seemed defensive about that topic probably because she knew she was losing control of even the most basic activities. I ordered an adjustable hospital bed with railings to be delivered the following week and set up a tentative schedule for the nurse.

As I walked the hospice officials to their car after our meeting, the nurse said that Leah could die at any moment and likely would do so within a week. She said Leah would probably fall asleep and not wake up.

That possibility sounded pretty good, at least when compared to a painful death in a conscious state.

When I returned to the house, Leah had already walked to the bedroom and was asleep.

On Thursday, the sun came out on a peaceful day, but Leah woke up uncomfortable and restless.

"I don't know why I'm so tired," she said, kicking the covers off the bed.

She got up and lay on the couch for a few hours. At one point, she pulled herself up and hobbled to the roll-top desk.

"Can I get something for you, Miss Leah?" I asked.

"I'm not an invalid," she snapped, and then nearly fell over a box.

I rushed to assist her and helped her back to the couch. I told her sternly that she could not put herself in danger of falling. She argued, but I interrupted her.

"This isn't open for debate," I said, raising my voice.

I reiterated what the hospice nurse told her about falling and warned that I wouldn't be able to leave her alone if she put herself at risk.

Leah continued to disagree, but I cut her off again.

"God damn it, stop arguing with me!" I shouted and left the room.

I took the dogs outside and sat on the patio. I cried, feeling anger, sadness, and guilt. As I petted the boys, I realized that for Leah to stop debating with me would be a sign that she had given up.

I returned to the living room and apologized. We hugged, and I helped her to the bedroom where she slept for the rest of the day.

Leah didn't suffer any significant pain during the week, just moderate discomfort when she woke up. She took her oral pain pills, and every few days I placed a new pain patch on her back. But everything changed on Friday.

I don't know why Nick thinks I'm going to die. . . . I'll feel better if I just lie down.

On Friday afternoon, Nick called and asked me to buy some food and bring it over to their house. Leah had requested organic chicken, but Nick said not to worry about it. When I arrived, Leah called me into the living room and asked if the chicken was organic. I told her it wasn't, and she said that it needed to be organic. "It's not that difficult," she said. "I do it all the time."

Nick took the dogs for a walk and I stayed with Leah. "I don't know why Nick thinks I'm going to die," she said, out of nowhere. I paused, not knowing what to say. Then I told her that Nick was concerned because she was sleeping so much. It was pretty clear that she was not accepting of the fact that she was dying.

(Nick and Leah's former graduate student, Jillian)

Our plan was for Leah to die at home, but, as we learned throughout this ordeal, plans don't always work out.

Leah slept most of Friday morning, but when she woke up and staggered onto the couch in the living room, she was more agitated than the day before. She expressed uncharacteristic frustration with me, even at the dogs.

She said she was hungry for a chicken salad, but I had not shopped for several days and the refrigerator was bare. I called Jillian and asked her to buy some food.

I hung up the phone and returned to the living room. Leah asked if the chicken was organic, as we had eaten more organic food during the past few years. I should have told her that it was organic, but I said I didn't know. She became upset and insisted that she would only eat organic chicken.

Jillian arrived with the food, and I asked her to stay with Leah while I took the dogs for a walk. I needed to clear my head and calm down. I didn't want to fight with Leah again, although she seemed determined to win one last argument.

When I returned, Jillian told me that Leah was really upset about the chicken and about the fact that I thought she was going to die.

Leah's aggravation continued into the evening. She sighed loudly and tossed and turned in bed.

At one point, she stood up and stumbled toward the bathroom. I guided her to the toilet and helped pull down her pajama bottoms. Before she sat down, two mushy globs of feces dropped to the floor. I stared at the sight for a moment, startled by the image, and surprised that anything could come out of her after she ate so little. When she finished, I helped her up and wiped her.

She also threw up several times. I called hospice, and a nurse said to give Leah oral antinausea medication. A few minutes later, Leah threw up the medicine, and I called hospice again.

The nurse asked whether Leah's vomit looked like coffee grounds.

I said it appeared to be mucus.

She told me that was a good sign and instructed me to go to the emergency pharmacy and get new antinausea medication that would dissolve in Leah's mouth.

I called Kimo, and asked him to get the drugs because I was not about to leave Leah.

Kimo agreed to pick up the meds, but then he called a half hour later and said there was a mix-up at the pharmacy and it would take another 45 minutes.

I called hospice again, and they apologized for the delay. They told me to hold on for the medicine.

While we waited, Leah's pain intensified. She threw up several times and moaned in obvious pain. Every second was excruciating.

I could clean up her vomit and wipe her butt, but I couldn't stop her suffering with the medication we had at home. The anti-nausea medication Kimo was getting would not relieve the pain she was experiencing at that point. I told Leah she needed to go to the hospital, but she resisted.

"I'll feel better if I just lie down," she said, dropping onto the bed after another messy trip to the bathroom.

I finally couldn't watch her suffer any longer. I called hospice one last time, and they agreed that Leah needed to be admitted to emergency. Kimo arrived with the meds a few minutes before the paramedics took her to the hospital.

That Friday night about 11 p.m., Nick called and said Miss Leah wasn't doing well and asked me to get some medicine for her. I got to their house about 1:30 in the morning, and it was obvious that the medication wasn't going to help her. She was in a lot of pain. The ambulance came to transport her, and they put her on a gurney. She had her eyes closed, and I walked over and held her hand. She did not even know I was there and had no energy at this point.

Nick said, "Miss Leah, Kimo's here. He's holding your hand."

Like she got power from some mystical force, she opened her eyes, turned, and looked at me, somehow managed to lift herself slightly up off the gurney, reached out for me, and gave me the biggest hug that I've ever had. At that moment, I knew it was no longer about her; it was about her telling me that things were going to be okay.

(Nick and Leah's friend and colleague, Kimo)

Leah was admitted to emergency around 2:00 a.m. on Saturday. Ironically, or perhaps fittingly, she was placed in the same cubicle where she received the initial diagnosis the year before. They hooked her up to a morphine drip, which relieved the pain, but made her more nauseous. She threw up mucus, blood, tissue, and other gunk that did indeed look like coffee grounds and smelled like Hawkeye with a really bad yeast infection. I stood vigil over her with a small plastic container, catching whatever I could of the bile that spewed from her mouth.

When a new shift came on duty near dawn, a doctor came in to check on Leah. He looked at her and then at me.

"I'm sorry about your mother," he said.

"She's my wife," I told him.

He apologized profusely, explaining that he did not have time to read the chart.

"Don't worry about it," I said. "She looks like my grandmother."

In actuality, she barely looked human.

Leah was admitted to a private room in the ward for terminally ill patients at 4 p.m., more than 12 hours after she entered the ER. I went home to feed the dogs, although my neighbor Dee-Dee took care of them from that point on as I stayed at the hospital.

Several friends visited Leah that evening and night. I told her whenever someone came into the room. She struggled to open her eyes, although she could not keep them open for more than a split second.

That night, Juliane pointed out that I was wearing my favorite Rasputin stout tee shirt from the North Coast Brewing Company. The "Never Say Die" motto on the back struck her as ironic, as I was coaching my wife to actually die. The next time I went home, I took off that shirt and vowed to never wear it again.

Leah gasped loudly throughout the night, and the duration between breaths became longer and longer, up to 35 seconds. I held her hand, stroked her hair, and said everything I could to help her die. I told her that I loved her, that I'd take care of the boys, that there wasn't anything left for her to do, that it wasn't her fault, that it was okay to go, to look for her mom.

But somehow she hung on.

On Sunday, Leah's condition deteriorated further. She barely acknowledged visitors, although Kimo takes pride that Leah opened her eyes briefly and partially mouthed a goodbye to him when he left.

Our friend Sylvia visited that afternoon and suggested that I bring in a CD player and play holiday music for Leah. I rushed home and returned with our portable CD player and several Christmas and choir CDs. Leah responded the most when I played choir music, especially a Sacramento Choral Society CD recorded from 2000 when Leah was a member of the choir. A soprano, Leah twitched her eyes and moved her mouth whenever the female sopranos sang. Even in a seemingly unconscious state, she somehow heard the music and sang along.

I stayed next to her all night long, unable to sleep as her gasping intensified and her tremors became more frequent. I said everything I could to help her to die. I even lied to her at midnight on December 13th and told her that it was my birthday. She had said that she would try to hang on for that date, which was the next day.

I continued to play her CDs, but then I wondered if that music was keeping her alive. Late that night I decided to play my music. I whispered in her ear that I was getting a CD from the car and asked her not to die in the next thirty seconds. I sprinted to the parking lot and retrieved "The Essential Bob Dylan." When I returned I serenaded her for the rest of the night, especially during the song "Not Dark Yet," which had become my theme song of the previous month because of the refrain, "It's not dark yet, but it's getting there." I played that song over and over, and Leah continued to hang on.

During one period of sleep-deprived delirium, I considered smothering Leah with a pillow. I yelled at God for not taking her sooner, but then the dark vestiges of my Catholic upbringing resurfaced and I realized it was Satan who was tormenting me with the ultimate paradox: the only way I could relieve my wife's suffering was to kill her, but then I'd be haunted with that memory for the rest of my life. I prayed, I cried, I swore, I sang, and I even laughed, fueled by adrenaline and feeling every possible emotion.

In the wee hours of Monday morning, I felt a moment of calm. Even though Leah gasped for breath and smelled horribly, the scene was eerily serene, even elegant. I did not feel a greater spiritual presence, but the moment itself was profound in its own right. I gazed around the room for several minutes and then summoned Leah's attention.

"Leah?" I said, and repeated her name several times until she partially responded. "I have to tell you something. I want you to know that I love you. I love you so much."

Leah twitched her eyes.

"Uv ü," she whispered, barely audible.

I kissed her forehead and wept.

By the time I got to the hospital, it was probably after eleven at night. Nick was by Leah's bedside, and he told her that I was there. She stirred a little, but didn't say anything. At that point, she was heavily medicated on morphine and coughing up a lot of blood and tissue. I spoke to her a little, but mostly spent my time trying to give what comfort I could to her and to Nick.

We talked about the irony—I guess that's the right word—of Nick being the first person to visit my wife and newborn daughter in the very same hospital just months before. One tries to say something comforting and wise in such circumstances, but what can be said at that point? My wife tells me that when her father died, the best thing that anyone said to her was that they can't possibly know how she must feel. I said that and brought Nick some food so that he could have some strength as he sat with Leah. After a while, I whispered some words of peace to her and then left.

(Nick and Leah's friend and colleague, Dave)

———————————————

At 6 a.m., Sylvia returned. She took one look at me and told me to go home and take a shower. I resisted, knowing that Leah could die at any moment, but then she could have died at any time during the previous week. I thought Leah might hang on for another day or two, so I decided to go home for a quick shower.

As I gathered my belongings, two nurses came in and said they wanted to turn Leah again to prevent bedsores. They started to move her and she became very distressed. She opened her eyes widely and craned her neck. In her withered condition and with bulging eyes and a stretched neck, she did not appear to be human. As ghastly and surreal as this might sound, she looked like E.T. from the Steven Spielberg movie.

I held her hand and told her it was okay, but she remained agitated even after the nurses left the room. Her breathing changed dramatically, shifting to what sounded like a higher octave, but in a minor chord.

"Something is different," I said.

Sylvia backed off and let me have privacy with Leah as I stroked her hair and coached her to die. I told her that it wasn't her fault, that I was so proud of her, and that she could do this. Her breathing slowed and her gasps shortened, until I could see only faint reflexes in her mouth and throat.

A few minutes past 7 a.m., Leah took one last microgasp and then became completely calm.

Sylvia approached and asked, "Is she gone?"

"I don't know," I said. "I've never done this before."

I put my finger on Leah's neck to feel for a pulse, and her throat quivered ever so slightly. We let her lie in peace for several additional minutes. She probably was dead for 5 minutes before I went to get a nurse.

I walked to the nurses' station and asked for help.

"Be right with you, honey," the nurse said as she filled out some paperwork.

"Take your time," I said calmly. "My wife just died and she's not going anywhere."

The nurse dropped her pen, stood up, and gave me her full attention.

"Are you okay?" she asked.

I told her I was fine and that I had been expecting Leah to die at any time for the last week. The nurse checked on Leah and called for a doctor.

Some nurses' aides came in to move Leah, to avoid bedsores—in more lucid moments later I realized the absurdity of needing to move someone so close to death—and it distressed Leah a lot. Her blue, blue eyes opened up wide, panicked, and she turned, not seeing anything in the room. Nick rushed to her other side, soothing her through words, stroking her hair, her arm, her hands, telling her how much he loved her, that it was okay to let go, reminding her that they had talked about everything, that "the boys" were okay.

I stepped back by then, not wanting to intrude, but not wanting to abandon Nick if he needed me. Each silence between breaths took longer, longer, with Nick softly talking to her the whole time, a murmur of loving words. Finally, there were long silences between the harsh, hard sounds of those last, final breaths. When she took her last breath, we just sat with her for a while, quiet, waiting.

(Nick and Leah's friend and colleague, Sylvia)

Kimo arrived shortly after Leah died and sat with me as I continued to hold Leah's hand. He said he would always remember Leah's clear blue eyes.

I told him her eyes were still crystal clear, a condition I never understood given what her body went through. I stood up and moved over Leah's body. I told Kimo to approach, and I propped open Leah's left eyelid with my finger and thumb.

"Look at how clear they still are," I said.

Kimo took a quick look at her and sat back down. I closed her eyelid and then he looked up at me.

"And you wouldn't look at your grandmother's body?" he said and smiled, a reference to when my paternal grandmother died and I refused to look at her body in the casket because I do not like the last memory of a loved one to be of their stiff cadaver in a box.

"Things have changed a little," I said and smiled.

A doctor came in around 8 a.m. to make the pronouncement of death. Kimo and I stayed with Leah until nearly 9:00 a.m., when the man from the crematorium came to take her body. He looked like a character from "The Sopranos."

"I'm sorry for your loss," he said softly.

Kimo helped me to my car and gave me one last long hug. I cried in his arms and then managed to drive home. I couldn't believe that she was actually gone.

11

Death Work

To: Leah Update List
From: nickt@csus.edu
Subject: Leah Update
Date: December 13, 2004

Hello All — Here is the news that no one wanted to hear, but everyone expected. Leah died earlier today at around 7:10 a.m. I was with her all night long until her death. She was not in pain, but was not conscious and seemed from time to time to struggle against the effects of the morphine drip. She also told me last week that she wanted to make it to my birthday (tomorrow) and she might have been holding on for that as well. At midnight last night, I whispered a thank-you for holding on for my birthday (I lied), and I told her that she could move on. Several friends visited her throughout the weekend, and I put the phone to her ear so she could hear wishes from family members. She died relatively peacefully this morning.

She will be cremated today. There will be a service at Carmichael Presbyterian Church later this week or weekend for any family and friends who wish to attend — I'll provide information once the date and time are confirmed.

In lieu of flowers, I ask anyone who wishes to contribute to donate to one of two funds that have been established in Leah's honor.... Please tell any friends and colleagues who know Leah about these funds, and feel free to forward this message to anyone.

Thank you all for your support, friendship,
and everything during this past year, especially
during the past couple months. Her death is a
huge loss for all of us, but her legacy will
live on.
    Take care. Love,
    nick

For my funeral, I would like to have Pastors Keith and/or Carol read Psalm
21 and then passages from John 14:1–7 and James 1:16–27. I also would
like the choir to sing the hymn "In This Very Room." That always made
me cry whenever we sing it. If they can play Barber's "Adagio for Strings"
over the speakers, that would be swell. That is one of my all-time favorites.
It is like the eternal unfolding, like a beautiful never-ending goodbye. It is
an exquisite piece of music. The e.e. cummings poem "I thank You God
for most this amazing" would be nice too.
    I wish that I could be there.

---

*I came over to Nick's house very soon after Leah had died. Leah
had asked me to take care of him, in ways that only I could, and
I did so. When I entered the home, there was a heavy feeling in
the air. It is difficult to describe. I don't remember the specifics
of our conversation, but Nick seemed to be acting normal.*

                    (Leah and Nick's friend and colleague, Diego)

You might think that immediately after a death there is a great sense
of relief, and there was a momentary one. But as soon as I got home,
I had a long list of things to do. I immediately sent out an e-mail to
the Leah Update List announcing the news of her death, and I called
her father and my mother to let them know. I called Leah's church to
make arrangements for the funeral. I called Kimo and asked him to
gather information about nearby hotels to send via e-mail to people
who would attend the funeral. I called the crematorium to confirm
that they had received her body and to schedule a time to pick up

her ashes. I called a colleague in journalism to see whether she could arrange for a nice obituary. I called another colleague who agreed to have a poster-sized photograph of Leah made for the funeral. I'm sure I did a few other things as well. And of course I fed my dogs.

About an hour or so after I arrived home, my colleague, Diego, came over to pick up a photograph of Leah for the poster. He gave me a hug and then stood back and looked me over.

"You don't look like your wife just died," he said.

I was totally sleep-deprived, but still on an adrenaline rush from Leah's death. "I'm not sure how one is supposed to look after his wife just died," I said, and I told him that I'd be okay.

Sometime that afternoon, I went to the bedroom, collapsed on the bed, and cried myself to sleep. I woke up a few hours later and couldn't fall back asleep, so I got up and looked through several photo albums in search of pictures of Leah to put on poster boards that a church official suggested I make for the reception after the funeral.

Kimo called that night and asked whether I wanted to come over to his house for my birthday the next day. I hadn't even thought about my birthday, apart from telling Leah on her deathbed that it was the day before. Normally, Leah and I went to the beach on my birthday, and I decided to go to the nearby Sonoma Coast for the day. I felt the need to escape, at least for part of a day.

The next day was a cool, windy one, but I took the boys to the beach in the van. I usually cut through Napa and Sonoma valleys, but the Highway 12 exit on I-80 was closed. A long line of cars had to take a detour at the following exit and use an alternate route.

A Highway Patrol officer stood on the street redirecting traffic as we idled along the detour. I asked him what the problem was.

"Fatality on Highway 12," he said matter-of-factly.

A chill went through my body. Somebody else would be making funeral arrangements for a loved one that week.

Ebbet, Hawkeye, and I finally arrived at Wright's Beach, a state park north of Bodega Bay with several campsites nearly on the beach. Winter storms had flooded much of the area, creating several large pools of salt water about 20 yards from the shoreline in what normally is a wide beach.

I parked the van in a site that was only partially flooded and took the boys on a walk. I dictated my thoughts into a tape recorder so I'd remember as many details as possible about the last few days at the hospital.

Wright's Beach is a very dangerous area. Waves break close to the shoreline, and there is a nasty riptide that can pull inexperienced beachcombers into the sea. A few adults, children, and/or dogs drown there every year. Even on a calm day, I never let the dogs run off leash at Wright's Beach.

The boys and I reached the southern point and turned around to head back to the campsite. I noticed two women and an unleashed dog about 100 yards away. One of the women and the dog were way too close to the shoreline.

I quickened my pace when I saw a large wave headed for the woman and the dog.

I screamed, "Watch out!"

The wave crashed on shore, and fortunately the woman and the dog were forced into one of the large pools of water inland. Otherwise they might have been swept into the ocean.

The dog quickly crawled out of the pool, but the woman flailed in the water. Her friend rushed to her aid, as the boys and I continued to run toward them.

By the time I arrived, the woman had struggled to her feet and was hip-deep in frigid water. She laughed, although her partner was not amused.

"What the hell is wrong with you?" I said with a tone of anger, mostly upset that the woman put her dog in danger. "You shouldn't let your dog run around at this beach."

"I come here all the time," the woman said and kept laughing.

"It isn't funny," her friend said, and walked away.

The boys and I walked away as well. I felt as if death and destruction were surrounding me.

I drove home late that afternoon and spent the evening looking through more Leah photographs.

The next day, I picked up Leah's ashes at the crematorium. An official advised me that there were bone fragments in the ashes because the company does not crush all the bones into powder. I signed a release form indicating I knew the laws regarding the distribution of human remains, which allow for the scattering of ashes on private property and in the ocean at least 500 yards from the coast. I said I planned to scatter her ashes on our property in Fort Bragg, although I didn't reveal my intention to also scatter her on the beach near our property.

That afternoon, I talked with the reporter writing Leah's obituary. I was pleased the obit would be published the next day, the day before her funeral.

I reached for the paper with anxiety the next morning. I knew Leah's story would be inside the Metro section, but I didn't expect to see a photo of her smiling face at the top right-hand corner on page one of that section. The caption read, "Leah Vande Berg, a professor at CSUS, has died."

I fell to my knees and wept. Although I knew the story would be there, the shock of seeing it in the newspaper was too much. After all, if it's in the paper, it must be true.

I read the article and wept. It was a lovely one, emphasizing Leah's passion for teaching.

In the afternoon, I went to a nearby mall to buy funeral pants and stopped in for lunch at a restaurant. Newspapers were all around, and I saw a woman reading Leah's obituary. I felt like screaming, "That's my wife!"

Instead, I ate a small salad in silence, barely maintaining my composure.

That night I made five posters with photos representing various phases of Leah's life. Every picture seemed to display her signature smile. I was mesmerized by the sheer joy of this woman. I could have made 50 posters that night.

I recalled when Leah and I made photo albums the nights after our dogs Rory Pooh, Wrigley, and Ragbrai died. We needed to see images of our beloved canines. I felt the same way about Leah, and I gazed at her photos until I feel asleep on the couch.

The funeral took place the next day. I arrived early, and an official took my posters and escorted me to the room where family members would gather. I was amazed, but not surprised, at how many people streamed into the church, including friends and colleagues from across the country.

In the family room, my parents and sisters met Leah's dad, stepmom, and brother. My mother had met Leah's brother and his family a month earlier, but no one else in our respective families had ever met. Someone said it wasn't the happiest occasion to meet, but everyone was cordial.

A church official escorted us inside the sanctuary, and I was blown away to see it filled to capacity with what Pastor Keith estimated to be more than 300 people. I smiled at several familiar faces, and I took a seat next to my father in the first row.

I looked up and saw Leah's smiling face on a huge poster at the front of the church. I stared into her blue eyes and welled up.

"Oh, wifey," I whispered. "Oh, Miss Leah."

She really was dead, and this really was her funeral.

I cried throughout the ceremony and remember very little of what happened. I do recall when Pastor Carol uttered the chilling words,

"Leah Vande Berg is dead." I remember Kimo getting a big laugh when he said that Leah loved me unconditionally, "which, if you know Nick, isn't easy." And I remember the choir singing, "In This Very Room."

I am so glad my colleague, Diego, videotaped the service. I watched it for the first time a few months later and realized what a beautiful funeral it was. Leah had planned it to perfection.

Afterward, everyone gathered in a hall for a brief reception. I was the unwitting celebrity, and a long line of people waited to pay respects, hug me, and wish me well.

Many friends had called or e-mailed to say they couldn't make it because of other commitments. I was too shell-shocked to take note of who wasn't there, but I will always remember the people that were there. I hugged and thanked almost all of them.

During the funeral, I was very focused on Nick and on Leah (her picture). I kept moving back and forth between the two of them, even though I could only see the back of Nick's head most of the time. I watched as his hand reached to his face. I knew he was wiping away tears. It made me cry. I wondered how I would handle the same situation. Not wanting to imagine it, but wondering.

I remember standing patiently at his side immediately after the funeral, waiting to hug him while he finished talking with the person before me. Feeling his strength and his intense sadness in one moment. Noticing how talkative he was, more than I had ever experienced with him before. It made sense, when later he told all of us in an e-mail that he was trying to embrace who Leah was and be more like her. The whole ceremony was a VERY beautiful tribute to her.

(Nick and Leah's friend, Patricia)

```
To: nickt@csus.edu
From: Harry
Subject: Love to you
Date: 12/19/04
```

Dear Nick:
    Your messages have been a blessing to all of
us graced by the friendship that you and Leah have
given us. I am very grateful for the final update
I just read. I've been thinking about you for
days. The memorial service was the last gift that
she gave. I sit here crying and smiling with the
knowledge that Leah's memory will live on in the
lives of so many.
Harry [Nick and Leah's friend]

After the reception I went home to feed the dogs. They had to eat, and I had to feed them. If I had kids, I would have had to get them ready for bed. Life continues, and immediately.

My department had scheduled our annual holiday party that night, during which we usually exchange silly "white elephant" gifts. The chair had suggested that we cancel the party, but I asked to gather to celebrate Leah's life. My colleague, Ray, and his wife graciously hosted a postfuneral reception at their home.

The gathering was wonderful. Our families met most of our friends, which showed them how much Leah was loved by so many people. It also showed them I had a huge support network and I would be okay.

Our friend, Thom, who had flown in from Columbus, Ohio, played his auto-harp and sang the song "Where I'm Bound." Other friends and colleagues, some of whom also had flown in from other states, sang along.

My Uncle Chuck leaned over and patted me on the knee.

"This is like an Irish wake," he said. "You're lucky to have so many friends. You're going to be fine."

I smiled and nodded in agreement, although I wasn't feeling very fine at that moment.

When Leah's dad, stepmother, and brother said they had to leave, I escorted them to the door. Leah's dad noticed I was fiddling with my wedding ring, which actually was *his* ring. Leah wanted to wear her deceased mother's wedding ring, and Morry graciously let me wear his wedding ring as my own.

I told Morry that Leah wanted me to give both wedding rings to her niece, Anna Leah, and I asked whether that was fine with him. He said yes, but told me I could wear it as long as I needed.

"How long are you supposed to wear it?" I asked.

"You're supposed to wear it for a year," Leah's stepmother said in what I heard as an evaluative tone. "That's what I did when my husband died."

"Well, Morry couldn't have worn his ring for a year because you were married less than a year after Norma died," I pointed out.

When I got home that night, I took the ring off and placed it on the window shelf in the kitchen, along with a cross that Leah kept on her desk.

I felt very strange not wearing that ring. I never took it off during our marriage, not even to play golf or garden. I stared at the indentation around my ring finger. It looked like a scar. I was scarred. The death of my wife had left an indelible mark on me.

The next few days are a blur. I paid several overdue bills, walked the dogs, and talked to various friends and relatives on the phone. I also went out to dinner with a couple graduate students and their husbands. They were very kind to ask, although it felt like a pity invitation. During the meal, I felt like one half of a picture.

To: nickt@csus.edu
From: susan
Subject:
Date: 1/21/05
        Dar nick, just wanted you to know that I think ofyou all thetime. It's just that thinking or speaking of you makesme think of leah, which makes me cry a lot and I'mjust not brave enough yet.still, when we walk the beaches with the mutts iremember so many happy times with the 4 of you. We arereally glad you were able to stay at our house. I hopewe can see you soon. i'm typing with only two fingers because the others are not very nimble, and it's getting tiresome, so i'll quit. please keep in touch.
love, susan
[Nick and Leah's friend, who died 3 weeks later from colon cancer]

My mom asked me to come home for Christmas, but I needed to be by myself during the holidays. Cal and Susan had offered me their house in Fort Bragg while they spent the holidays in Santa Barbara. Getting away from Sacramento for a while sounded very good, and fortunately I had 5 weeks off before the spring semester would begin. I left for Fort Bragg on Christmas evening, figuring correctly there would be few cars on the road.

On the drive up the coast, I thought about whether I should keep the land in Fort Bragg or sell it and find a new place, perhaps in Big Sur. But the moment I arrived in Fort Bragg, I knew it was not just "our" dream to live, it was *my* dream as well.

The next day, it rained pretty hard. I scattered about one quarter of Leah's ashes under a tree on our land, along with the ashes of her dogs, Rory Pooh and Ragbrai. As the ashes fell, I couldn't believe that was what remained of my wife. I wanted to go to the beach for a second scattering, but decided to wait for a sunny day to do that.

Afterward, I went to lunch at our favorite brewpub and sat down at the bar. The couple next to me struck up a conversation and asked whether I was from around here.

"No, but my wife and I bought land here a few years ago," I said.

"Oh, you're married," the woman said.

I paused, and then told them she died a week earlier.

"Oh my God," the woman exclaimed. An awkward pause followed, and the couple left within minutes, although they were looking at a menu. I guess they thought my head—or my heart—was about to explode.

A few minutes later, a 20-something guy wearing a Giant's cap sat next to me. He looked over and asked whether I lived there.

"No, but we own some land here," I said, and then paused.

"You and your wife?" he asked.

I told him my wife died a week ago.

"Oh, man," he said, and within minutes he left the bar.

After those encounters, I told anyone I met that my wife died several months ago. After January 1, I said my wife died "last year."

Upon hearing that, people expressed sympathy, but did not run for their lives.

After about a week, I could tell people that "I" had purchased land there. I realized that although I felt like a neon sign of despair, to others who didn't know me I was just a regular guy who could engage in regular conversations, at least if I didn't say my wife just died.

Leah and I were always cordial to anyone we met in Fort Bragg, but we were happy camping by ourselves with the dogs and spending a little time with Cal and Susan. But if I really was going to live there, I thought I should develop my own network of friends there. One night at a bar in Mendocino, a local named Greg, who goes by "G.B.," and his fishing buddy, Rich, adopted me after I told them my wife had died a few months earlier. I hung out with them that night and on several other occasions, and I met their circle of friends.

On New Year's Eve, I went to the Caspar Inn to hang out with G.B. and his friends and to listen to live music. It had rained for several days and the ground was saturated, and I parked my van in a ditch and got stuck in mud. When the wheels spun, I slammed my fist into the steering wheel and yelled an obscenity. But then I took a deep breath and realized that I had just been through the worst experience of my life, and so getting stuck in the mud was not that big a deal.

"What's the worst that'll happen?" I asked myself. I might have to take a cab home and get the van towed in the morning. But I also thought I could find some guys to push it out. I told myself it would work out and went into the club.

When G.B. was about to go home several hours later, I told him about my predicament. He said he knew a guy who needed a ride to Fort Bragg who might find some friends to get me out of the mud in exchange for a ride.

I tracked the guy down and made the offer. He agreed, found his friends, and within minutes my van was out of the mud. I gave him a ride to Fort Bragg and returned to the bar until it closed.

We met Nick at Patterson's Pub in Mendocino one night. We could tell he was hurting, it didn't really matter why. We took him on a tour of Mendocino bars. I ended up making a new friend.

(Nick's friend, G.B.)

While in Fort Bragg, I also reached out to Leah's and my friends. Leah was my link to most other people in our lives, except for my buddy, Kimo. She was the one who called our friends, who insisted on throwing parties, who made me go to other people's parties. I always prided myself on being a bit of a loner. But I knew I couldn't grieve alone.

I had brought our address and phone book with me and called many people, some of whom I had never called in my life. A few were surprised when they answered and it was the guy whose wife had just died, but everyone was supportive.

It felt good to initiate contact with people, although I did run up a big long-distance bill.

I also thought it would be nice to send shells from the cove where I scattered Leah's ashes to her friends and relatives. But I have always lived by the philosophy that no one should take more than one shell from a beach. I get irritated when parents allow their children to pillage buckets of shells and sand dollars. They usually end up in a box or a backyard anyway, and then there are fewer shells on the beach for others to see.

But this time I went to the Leah cove and hoarded a boatload of shells. Most were flat shells that could fit in a card, although I had to pay 12 cents additional postage even for the flattest ones. I selected bigger and rounder shells for close friends and relatives and wrapped them in plastic and sent them in padded envelopes.

Unfortunately, many of them broke in transit, and I ended up sending broken shells. I suppose the pieces symbolized my broken life.

Kimo came up to visit for a few days, no doubt to check up on me. He arrived at night, and the next day I took him to the Leah cove and let him scatter some of Leah's ashes there.

Leah had initially wanted half of her ashes scattered in Fort Bragg and half on her mother's grave in Iowa, but during the last week of her life we discussed other possible scatterings. She liked the idea of scatterings on our campus with department colleagues and at the University of Iowa with her former professors.

"It doesn't matter to me," she said one night about 2 weeks before her death. "I won't be around anyway."

She told me to do whatever I thought was appropriate.

As I watched Kimo scatter her ashes and experience his Leah moment, I decided to have several scatterings to let other friends and relatives have their Leah moments. Knowing it is illegal to scatter ashes in public places, I filled a plastic bag with sand from the cove that I mixed in with her ashes to give me plausible deniability in case a police officer or park ranger ever caught me scattering her ashes with a group of people. I could say we were doing a "symbolic scattering."

After 4 weeks in Fort Bragg, I felt nearly normal. I had made an effort to go out and listen to music, to go to art shows, and to meet people, and it paid off. I met a dozen or so people and had started a new network of friends. I didn't feel like a walking beacon of grief and despair. I was even getting excited about my new life. With the life insurance money, two small pensions, and our 403B investments, I could build my house in Fort Bragg and retire much earlier than I had intended. I still wanted Plan A, but Plan B was looking pretty damn good.

I actually felt better than after my divorce when I believed I had made a huge mistake and wondered whether we might ever get back together again. In Leah's case, there was no second-guessing, and there was a clear sense of closure.

I could have stayed in Ft. Bragg for the rest of my life. But I had to go back to work in Sacramento.

Leah had asked me to keep an eye on Nick and make sure he was all right. That was one of the biggest motivations to go up to Fort Bragg to see him. He and the boys seemed to be doing fine. We played golf and took walks along the beach. One night we stayed up until around 4:00 a.m. listening to music, taking turns picking our favorite song off of all of his CDs.

Nick said he had met a bunch of people up there. One night we were looking through the windows of some place where people were dancing the tango. A guy came out that Nick had met, but when Nick said hello to him the guy didn't remember Nick. I loved teasing him about that.

When I scattered Leah's ashes on the beach, I said goodbye to her and reflected on her life. I was very sad that she was gone, but I was also happy to have spent time with one of the most amazing people I've ever met in my life.

(Leah and Nick's friend, Kimo)

The moment I arrived back in Sacramento, there was another pile of death work to complete. I needed to make copies of Leah's death certificate, to fill out forms to receive the life insurance benefits and my share of her pension, and to notify dozens of organizations about her death, including the social security office, credit card companies, the bank, the utilities, and others. I also had to prepare syllabi for my classes and get ready for a new semester.

Unlike Fort Bragg, where no one knew about Leah's death unless I told them, every one of my friends and colleagues in Sacramento knew about it. After those 4 weeks, I felt nearly normal, but now I reverted back to being a grieving widower.

I was reminded of that status when a friend whose wife had died from breast cancer a few years earlier called to check on me.

"How are you doing?" he asked.

"All in all, I think I'm doing okay," I said.

"Well, I know you're not okay and you won't be okay for a long time," he replied.

An awkward pause followed as I took a deep breath. I told him I knew he was trying to help, but saying I would not be okay for a long time wasn't helpful. I asked him to tell me what he had gone through. He said he was reluctant to do so because he said he made several mistakes during his grief. I asked him to tell me what those mistakes were so that I might avoid them. It was the most instructive conversation I ever had about grief.

My friend said he didn't like to cry, so he did not look at his wife's picture for several months. He said he and his two teenage children didn't talk about her death for a few months because it was too emotional. He said people called him for a couple weeks after his wife's death, but then stopped calling, and he became upset that no one was calling. He said his wife wanted to be scattered at Yosemite, but years later they still hadn't done so because it would be too emotional. He said he isolated himself and avoided contact with people and did not talk openly about his grief.

Then he admitted that *2* years after her death, he had to go to therapy because he had not truly grieved for his wife.

My friend's disclosure about his grief experience was a wonderful gift. I realized that in many ways I had not really even begun to grieve, and he provided a list of pitfalls that I tried to avoid.

I did not have a problem with crying, but I realized I had not cried in a few weeks. I knew that as a former college athlete crying did not come naturally to me, so the next day I purchased sad music, including Bruce Springsteen's "The Rising." Springsteen recorded the CD following the September 11 attacks, and it is an especially powerful one with some brutally sad songs. For example, the track, "You're Missing," includes the refrain: "You're missing when I shut out the lights, you're missing when I close my eyes, you're missing when I see the sunrise." Another one, "My City of Ruins," includes the verse: "Now there's tears on the pillow, Darling, where we slept. You took my heart when you left. Without your sweet kiss my soul is lost my friend. Tell me how do I begin again."

Those songs definitely helped me to cry. But after playing them for a few days, I couldn't stop crying. The challenge during the next several weeks, then, became getting through those songs without crying.

My friend's admission that he hadn't discussed his grief with many people motivated me to maintain the openness with which Leah and I approached her cancer and death during my grief. I expected to become more private about my grief after her very public death, but I decided to continue to be open about my feelings and even post an occasional message about my grief to the Leah Update List.

My friend's disclosure about isolating himself also motivated me to become more social in grief than I was in marriage. I had reached out to others during Leah's illness and death and during my month in Fort Bragg, but I assumed I would slip back into my familiar routine as a "hermit crab." Instead, I continued to reach out to others, especially the friends and relatives in Leah's huge network.

The absolute best advice my friend gave me was to not let other people bother me. He said that during his grief people said all kinds of things, some of which were not very helpful.

People do indeed say dumb things to patients with a terminal illness and to widows and widowers, although I'm sure they mean well. I can't tell you how tiring it was to hear people say, "You must feel horrible."

I was tempted to say, "I was feeling pretty good until you mentioned it," but I would nod and half-smile.

Another favorite: "This must be the worst time in your life."

I wanted to say: "No, the weekend of my wife's death was the worst time of my life. The second worst time was when I saw my best friend almost burn to death when I was a kid. My divorce was the third. Getting zits in high school wasn't fun either."

But again, I would just nod and half-smile.

I understand that in our culture we are not taught how to interact with someone who has cancer or has just lost a loved one. In my opinion, the best thing you can say to someone who has gone through this experience is, "How are you?"

But unlike the ritualistic greeting, "How's it going?", you really need to care how they are doing, and you really need to listen to what they say.

I wanted to take a leave from teaching that semester, but I was told I might have to postpone my sabbatical if I did. I thought, "What would Leah do?" She taught with cancer, and she most certainly would teach during grief. So I bucked up and went back to work.

I began my classes as usual, but I knew it would be the most unusual semester of my career. Many students knew that my wife had died a month earlier, so I felt the need to acknowledge it. I told them that my wife would have continued to work, as she had done during her illness.

I was very aware that others were observing me. I recognized my status as an unwitting role model, just as Leah was during her cancer. So just as Leah had taught others how to live with cancer and die with dignity, I felt a responsibility to teach my students, friends, and relatives how to grieve with joy and continue to live.

Once classes started, teaching was relatively easy. The hardest part was coming home on Thursday evening after my last class for the week. Leah and I would always pop open a bottle of wine to celebrate. The house felt so empty without her. The dogs were there, but they didn't talk back, and they couldn't drink wine with me.

But I was determined not to isolate myself and not to grieve alone.

12

Communal Grief, Joyous Grief

I stopped in Sacramento to see Leah and Nick on the way home from a leadership conference in Palm Springs. There were several fantastic and inspirational speakers there, including Former Russian President Mikhail Gorbachev and Benazir Bhutto, former prime minister of Pakistan.

The worst speaker was Malcolm Gladwell, who wrote "The Tipping Point." Ironically, despite his ennui during his presentation, he gave me insight into Leah. He described, from his book, a type of person he called a "Connector." And it was spot on Leah. Connectors are those rare people who know and have time for everyone, from the mail man, associates, to ordinary people in the routine of life, even the butcher. Leah knew the grocery store clerks and asked about their families while checking out. She cared about the details of other lives in a way that I had never seen before. She knew the birthdays of many, maybe hundreds. Somehow she had a magical social gift.

When I walked back into their house and the card boa was still draped across the room, only to have grown over the course of the year, all I could think of was Gladwell's description. Leah was indeed a "Connector."

(Leah and Nick's friend, Laurie)

Dear Mr. Nickers,
Never ever forget that I love you with all my heart!
Wifey, Leah

(Card from Leah that I found in a drawer after her death)

During the spring semester, I set out on a mission to have as many Leah celebrations as possible with the many friends in her networks. I wanted to honor her life and legacy, but I also knew the various people in her life needed to grieve as well.

The first event was an informal scattering with the eight people who visited Leah in the hospital that final weekend. I called them "the gang of eight," a nickname that originally referred to the eight people hired by our department in 1990, including Leah and me. I asked my gang of eight to meet me on campus at a place near the American River, where Leah and I used to walk the boys.

The only time when eight busy people could meet was late afternoon on the first Friday of the new semester. Rain poured down that entire January afternoon, and as I pulled into campus, a rare lightening bolt struck the Sacramento Valley several miles away. I didn't want to reschedule the scattering, though, and I hoped everyone would come.

One by one they arrived, wearing raincoats and holding umbrellas. Most of them commented on the harsh weather, although as we milled around the rain lessened a bit.

When the final person arrived, we gathered in a circle. And before our eyes the rain stopped and a rainbow appeared.

Because this was my first public scattering, I wasn't sure what to say. I told the gang I had mixed in sand from the Leah cove because scattering ashes in a public place was against the law, but I assured them there was enough of Leah to make it legitimate. I also warned them that there were some small bone fragments in the mix.

I wanted to say a prayer because Leah was so devout. I told the gang that Leah always said a prayer before we ate formal meals, and early in our marriage her prayers were so long that dinner was cold by the time she finished. I said I had instituted a 1-minute-or-less policy for her dinnertime prayers; in the spirit of that practice and because of the weather, I offered a very brief prayer. I began with the words Leah used to start all of her prayers: "Dear good and gracious God." I followed it with, "Thank you for Leah, and thank you for our friends."

Each person took a handful of the mixture and scattered it in the grass and/or on the bushes overlooking the river. Afterward, a few people offered their thoughts on her life and/or on that weekend in the hospital.

In retrospect, I regret not inviting other friends from campus, especially the few who visited Leah at home during the last week of her life. But I didn't want to make the scattering an entire department function especially because I did not have permission from university officials. I also didn't know which people to include and exclude. I felt a profound bond with the people who went to the hospital on the final weekend, so they were my "gang of eight."

I wish I had brought the dogs, but they had already participated in two scatterings at the Leah cove in Fort Bragg.

I feel privileged to have been a part of the Leah scattering on campus. That's one of my strongest residual feelings: I was honored to be included. The people who were there are some of the most caring, loving people I know. It was nice to share the moment with them.

It was strange, too, though. I think most death rituals like scattering ashes occur in family settings, and my family has never done that. My experiences have been burials; even when my mom was cremated, we buried the remains. So this was not something I was familiar with personally, although it seemed fine to me conceptually—I wasn't weirded out by the thought, or anything. I think the strangeness came from two things: first, that there wasn't some sort of ceremony or specific ritual to follow, almost as a guidebook for what to expect, and second, that this was not a family gathering, which is the context I'm used to.

But it was also magical. I'll never forget how hard it had been raining, and how we had all come together in a rough circle when Catherine said, "Look! There's a rainbow!" Sure enough, a spectacular rainbow appeared on the scene. I like to think Dr. Miss Leah was responsible. Magical!

(Leah and Nick's friend and colleague, Chris)

The first 2 to 3 weeks of the semester dragged on. There were many lonely nights and moments of deep despair as I continued to listen to Springsteen and other sad songs. But I also tried to stay active by walking the dogs and getting back into tennis. And I forced myself to go out for live music or art shows once every week or two, often with my colleague, Josh.

In February, Josh accompanied me on "Second Saturday," the night of the month when art galleries in Sacramento host receptions.

Josh was still inside one gallery when I walked out and saw a former Sac State official. She greeted me warmly, expressed her condolences, and introduced me to a friend of hers that, as she said, "suffered a similar loss."

I said hello to the woman and asked how she was doing.

"Not very well," she answered quickly. She told me that she doesn't like to cry, so she did not look at his picture for a long time. She said she had bottled up her feelings and still wasn't dealing well with his death. She said she was angry, bitter, and depressed, and was going to therapy, but therapy was not going well either.

I asked when her husband died.

"Three years ago," she said.

I suppressed my surprise and offered a comforting smile.

"When did your wife die?" she asked.

"Two months ago," I said.

The woman scowled. "Then what are you doing here?" she asked.

"Umm," I stammered, caught off guard by her evaluative tone. "I'm living," I said and forced a smile. I told her that others who've had similar experiences suggested that I stay active, so I was biking, playing tennis, and going to art shows.

The woman shook her head.

"Well, a year from now you're going to have a complete break-down just like I did," she said and turned away.

I was shocked at the widow's reaction, but it reminded me that people handle grief very differently. And someone who doesn't handle it well does not necessarily want to hear about someone who does.

Later that month, the Western States Communication Association convention was scheduled to take place in nearby San Francisco. Because Leah would have been a vice president at that conference, I wanted to make it an extra special one in her honor.

```
To: Friends of Leah
From: nickt@csus.edu
Subject: Leah Update
Date: 1/26/2005
     Hello Friends of Leah — I would like to invite
you to a Leah scattering at WSCA on Saturday,
2/19 at 3:00 p.m. at China Beach, south of the
Presidio.... I thought China Beach would be an
```

appropriate place as Leah won the B. Aubrey Fisher
award for an article in the *Western Journal
of Communication* that she did on the TV show
"China Beach."

I don't know whether all of you are coming to
Western or if you'll arrive in time to attend, or
even if you want to attend such a gathering. But
if you want to come and will be there in time,
you are welcome....

Leah was loved by so many people at Western
that if I made this a convention event probably
more than 100 people would attend. But this is
meant to be a private ceremony for the still-
quite-large number of people who were close to
Leah and/or are close to me.... Thus, please do
not forward this e-mail to anyone and please
do not invite people who you see at the
convention to this ceremony.

However, I do not want to exclude any people
who were close to Leah (and I don't know everyone
at WSCA who was close to her, as she went to a
lot of meetings and parties while I just go to
a lot of parties). So please e-mail me privately
if you think I have excluded anyone, and I'll
follow-up with an invitation for them.

Thanks. Hope you can make this gathering.
Take care,
nickt

Because it was only a 2-hour drive from Sacramento to San Francisco,
I had the luxury of bringing things I could not bring to a convention if I had taken a plane. I really wanted to make this conference a
celebration of Leah's life, but I knew that people might feel the need
to leave me alone. To counter that possibility, I brought beer, wine,
hard liquor, and plenty of snacks, intending my room to be party
central. Who, after all, would turn down the opportunity to get free
booze and food?

I also brought the remainder of Leah's clothes, hats, and jewelry
that I hadn't sent to her niece, Anna Leah. I packed over a dozen hats
and many scarves, gloves, pins, and other items. Most of the stuff was

for women, although there were a few things that Leah's male friends could take, such as an Anchor Steam Beer pin that our friend Harry took.

When I pulled my overstuffed Subaru into the unloading area of the hotel, the head bellman frowned.

"All this stuff isn't going to your room, is it, sir?" he asked.

I told him my wife was an officer of the association and that she had died of cancer 2 months earlier. I said I wanted to host a reception for her and give her belongings to her friends.

He snapped his fingers, and two assistants instantly appeared and hauled all of the stuff to my room, needing three pull carts to do so.

My room looked like a miniature Turkish bazaar or Moroccan souk. I set up a full bar and a CD player, hung Leah's clothes in an open closet, and placed her hats, scarves, and other items everywhere.

When friends visited the room, I asked them to take an item. Most women immediately said, "I couldn't possibly take Leah's stuff," but 5 minutes later they were holding up hats and scarves in the mirror asking each other if it matched their outfits.

I also delivered a bunch of Leah's belongings to the room of the Sacramento State grad students. They had rented a suite to host parties in Leah's honor. In their room was the poster-sized photo of Leah from the funeral.

Throughout the conference, people hugged me and asked me how I was coping. Some uttered the all-too-familiar, "you must feel horrible" and "you must be having a hard time." My response to them probably sounded strange because I told them I was enjoying grieving for Leah. When I told one acquaintance, "I'm having a blast grieving for Leah," she looked at me like I was crazy.

I'm sure many people at the conference did think I was crazy or at least in denial, but I knew there was a relatively brief window when I could grieve intensely for her—talk about her, cry openly, share her belongings, arrange public scatterings—and I consciously took advantage of that window. I also thought about how joyously and lovingly Leah lived her life. I knew I could never be Leah, but I could be more Leah-like and show people that I was going to live my life in a more kind, loving, and joyous way.

Most of the people in Leah's network supported me with kindness and compassion. I felt so much love at that conference, but I also knew I was helping them grieve and deal with their loss as well.

There were many great moments. At the convention luncheon, Leah received the Distinguished Service Award, the highest honor given to members who make significant contributions to the association. I accepted the award on her behalf, and I told the audience how much Leah loved the association and thanked them for loving her. I received a standing ovation while I hugged members on the dais.

The association also named the debut paper award after Leah, an award given to a first-time presenter at the conference, usually a student. Fittingly, that year's recipient happened to be one of Leah's former students, Sheryl.

I had been told that my paper was one of the top debut papers, but I had no idea that I would receive the award. I almost didn't go to the luncheon because my sister-in-law wanted me to do something with her.

When they announced my name, I barely made it up there because I was so emotional. It was so special and humbling to receive that honor because Leah was so special to me. She encouraged me to continue with my education, and she always supported me. The mentorship she provided was incredible.

I miss her so much, but there are moments when I still feel her presence. One day I was walking my dog along the American River where Leah and Nick walked the boys, and I saw a coyote. She stopped and looked at me, and we stared at each other for a long time. I think she was there for a reason, to encourage me, like Leah always did.

(Leah's friend and former student, Sheryl)

For me, the highlight of the convention was the scattering at China Beach. About 20 close friends and colleagues attended despite pouring rain.

I began with my brief scattering prayer, and then each person took some of the ash-sand mixture from the brass container. I thought people would scatter her ashes and quickly return to the shelter of their cars, but most stayed for about a half hour in the rain. People walked around the beach by themselves and had their Leah moments.

One of Leah's former graduate students, Rona, brought a beautiful lei that finally made it out to sea after being pushed back ashore by the waves.

I noticed that one of Leah's other former students, however, did not take any of Leah's ashes. Earlier she told me that she was not dealing well with Leah's death, and Leah had expressed concern to me about her and asked me to help her. I walked over to the former student and offered the container, but she shook her head.

"I don't want to cry," she said.

"Look around," I said. "Everybody is crying." I looked at the sky. "Even the angels are crying."

"I'm not ready for closure yet," she said.

I told her closure was not a water faucet and that the scattering wouldn't offer complete closure. I asked her to take some of Leah's ashes, but she still refused. I was very sorry for her because all of Leah's close friends except her participated in this wonderful ceremony. This former student chose to isolate herself, which seemed to me to be another example of how she was not dealing well with the loss and how she was making Leah's death about her, rather than about Leah and Leah's friends.

My biggest regret was that I forgot to invite Leah's cousin who lived in the city. I was in my convention mode and just didn't think about it.

To Leah's scattering I brought a bright purple dendrobian orchid lei to throw into the ocean to honor her and say goodbye. This is a Hawaiian tradition of paying tribute to a loved one, of saying goodbye and wishing a hui hou, or until we meet again.

Many people showed up and Nick was there, shepherding us down the beach and looking strong. I handed Nick the lei and asked if he would throw it into the ocean. The lei, however, would not drift out to the ocean. It kept coming back. Nick and I laughed. He kept hurling it out there, and it would slide back. We laughed and he eventually got it out there.

Once I saw the lei in the ocean, I spent a few quiet moments talking to her. I whispered, "Oh Leah. I miss you, we all do. I don't know what I will do without you and how I will move on. I love you so much and I will make sure Nick is okay. Stay with me, stay with me."

I walked away from the scattering ironically wishing that Leah were there, to see her friends come and say goodbye, to hear the laughs and the memories, to know that her life will always be remembered and cherished and that we will never forget her.

(Leah's former student and their friend, Rona)

The day was rainy, dreary, and even a tad cold, and somehow that seemed fitting. I wonder if a sunny day would have seemed similarly fitting. Perhaps. But this day seemed a better fit for my mood.

For me, the scattering of ashes was mostly about grieving, saying goodbye, and somehow trying to make sense out of something so seemingly senseless.

I took some of the ashes—oh how eerie that seemed. This was Leah—no, not Leah—but something that represented the last tangible part of Leah. Now I would take this last piece of what remained of her physical presence and be part of scattering this back to the greater universe. I stood there trying to understand our connection with that world—my connection, Leah's connection, Leah's and my connection, my connection to the collection of people assembled—Leah's connection to the collection—the collection's connection to the larger universe—and the thoughts numbed my brain. It was not something I could understand or articulate. Yet, I felt it powerfully. I stood there on the shore, looking out to sea simply feeling. In the midst of death, I felt alive, connected and somehow okay.

My husband Peter called me over to share a beautiful starfish and told me he had scattered his part of Leah amongst the starfish. He too was feeling the larger connection.

We drove back to the hotel, and Nick invited us to his room to take something of Leah's that he brought for all of us. My eyes immediately landed on a beautiful gold starfish—a pin that whenever I wear it, others comment upon it. I felt as though Leah had purchased it for me to wear as a lasting reminder of our connection to each other and to things so much greater than us. Leah's ashes, the starfish, the starfish pin, my love of the pin—it all came together to wrap me in a bond that transcends the physical. The starfish is the reminder to me that in death we find life and that with life we encounter death. It's a circle that eludes our sensemaking, but fully enwraps our being. Whenever I wear the pin—and I do so frequently—I feel Leah, our circle, *and life's fullness and pain. It's one circle that no matter how we struggle cannot be broken.*

(Leah and Nick's friend, Jan)

I did not want that convention to end. Leah's memory was very much alive there, and all of her friends could feel her presence. I knew I would feel so much joy with our friends there and that I would feel sorrow when I returned to an empty house.

But home I went.

A month later, Leah's former choir director, Don, who had orchestrated the Christmas carol concert for Leah in our cul de sac announced that the Sacramento Choral Society would dedicate the opening concert of the Spring 2005 season to Leah. The performance took place at the Sacramento Convention Center theatre and featured Haydn's "Creation." Leah was a soprano in the large choral group for several years.

I received several complimentary tickets and was joined by my Aunt Robyn and her husband Ed, Kimo, and Jillian and Juliane, the two grad students who helped me take care of Leah during the last few months of her life.

I expected the concert to be hard for me, knowing I would see the chorus and not see Leah. But I was completely unprepared for what happened during the first half of the performance.

I had not listened to choral music since the weekend of Leah's death, when I played the CDs in the hospital. I appreciate choral music from an artistic standpoint, but rarely listen to it, preferring blues, jazz, and reggae. When the chorus kicked in, especially the female sopranos, I unexpectedly flashed back to that horrible weekend in the hospital. My friends and relatives thought I was tearing up because I missed Leah, but in fact I was reliving the nightmare of her death. I listened in agony during that first half and was very relieved when intermission came.

I told Kimo I needed some fresh air and started to walk toward the aisle. Just then a man walked down the stairs wearing a Rasputin Stout Ale tee shirt from the North Coast Brewing Company in Fort Bragg. I had not seen that shirt since I retired my own after Leah's death.

I nearly lost control. I shouted, "Stop that man!"

The man saw I was yelling at him and rushed out of the auditorium.

Kimo settled me down, and then I left the building. I took several deep breaths and wondered whether I would be able to return for the second half. I thought I might never be able to listen to choral music again without reliving her death.

But one of the lessons I tried to implement during my grief was to confront my emotions head on, just as Leah always did. I didn't want to avoid choral music for the rest of my life and break down every time I happened to hear it. I reluctantly came back for the second half, although I sat closer to the aisle in case I needed to leave again.

When the chorus kicked in after intermission, I took a few deep breaths and held on. It wasn't easy at first, but after 20 or so minutes, I envisioned Leah singing with the group and remembered how much joy that music gave to her. By the end of the performance, I was smiling and filled with joy.

Similar feelings were stirred up the following month when Leah's church dedicated a choir performance to her at a Sunday service. I hadn't been inside that church since Leah's funeral, and I knew it too would be emotional.

The moment I walked into the sanctuary, I recalled seeing the poster of her smiling face 4 months earlier. I tried to maintain my composure, but I lost it during the choir's performance. I sat as still as I could while tears rolled down my face. The person sitting next to me slowly slid away.

But, again, I confronted my emotions head on, and by the time the service ended, I was smiling with joy, grateful that Leah had such supportive friends at her church and that she was still being honored.

Several members of the church choir performed at the end of the campus celebration of Leah's life that month, where Leah's university friends and colleagues spoke about working with her. After that service, I sent a check to the church and requested that the money go specifically to the choir. It was a nice amount, but a small percentage of the money Leah donated to the church every year.

From nearly 15 years back, I can still remember the first real conversation with my friend, Leah. I don't remember what we talked about, but I do remember she seemed like the most charming person I had ever met. . . . Charming means captivating, and what captivated me most of all was her smile. I think it was her smile that most clearly conveyed her spirit. What a smile! The sun even on its most electric mornings has never conveyed more warmth than that smile. . . .

And as that sunny smile told me right from the start, she would be from first to last, my friend. And from our first meeting to our last one, she never failed to add her sunshine to my life, just as she, like the sunlight, offered it to all of us. . . .

(Leah and Nick's friend, Steve, from her campus service)

For Easter weekend, I went to Santa Cruz to attend my cousin Tom's gallery show. Tom is an artist, and his work was being featured at the downtown exhibit. Because many family members would be in attendance, I brought the container of Leah's remaining ashes in case we had time for a scattering.

At a family party on Easter Sunday, I told relatives I had brought Leah's ashes with me and invited everyone to go to the bluffs overlooking the ocean in La Selva Beach, just a few blocks from my cousin's house. About 15 relatives and friends joined me for yet another rainy day scattering.

The wind howled, and at times the rain seemed to fall horizontally. We huddled together, I said my scattering prayer, and relatives took ashes and had their Leah moments.

On the way back to Tom's house, one of my cousins said that "this" was going to happen to all of us, meaning death.

I added that what I was going through—the death of a spouse—would probably happen to half of them. After all, unless both spouses die in a car wreck or plane crash, one spouse almost always dies before the other one.

My relatives looked around at each other, no doubt wondering who would die first in their respective marriages.

At that moment, I realized I was the first one in my extended family to be widowed. I was not only serving as a role model to my students, but to my family as well.

I was not looking forward to seeing Nick without Leah. I think it is difficult for people to approach a widower, especially one as

*young as Nick was. But he was so gracious and serene, I felt
at ease.*

*The scattering at La Selva Beach was mystical. I had no
idea Nick had brought Leah along on the trip. I was sitting in the
yard looking at the clouds churning overhead thinking, "Wow a
storm is coming," and my brother Patrick saying the sky looked
different and that he couldn't remember seeing it like this. Soon
after, Nick said he had to leave and we were going to the beach
to scatter Leah's ashes.*

*The weather really started to kick up as we all headed to
the cliffs. Penny opened her umbrella and it immediately turned
inside out. Everyone arrived at the cliffs, and we all took a bit
of Leah and turned our backs to the wind.*

*"Fly with the wind Leah, Fly with the wind,"
I said.*

*Soon after, the storm kind of calmed down and blew away.
Very interesting.*

(Nick's cousin, Cathy)

People who have experienced the death of a spouse say it takes at
least a year to grieve because during the year after the death you go
through every possible anniversary—the anniversary of the diagnosis,
of the death, of the birthday, of the wedding anniversary, and others.
For me, our wedding anniversary was the worst.

We were married on July 20, and the first anniversary after her
death would have been our 20th anniversary. In our culture, round
numbers seem to make dates more meaningful, and 20 years of marriage would have been a very special celebration.

I took the boys to Fort Bragg, as Leah and I always did on our
anniversary. I arrived the evening before and ate at our favorite brewpub. I camped in the van on our land.

The next morning, I went to the Leah cove. It was foggy, but not
cold. I reflected on life without Leah. I sat on a big piece of driftwood
and wept. I missed her so much I ached. I had not had a good cry for
a while, but afterward I felt drained, rather than cleansed.

I could not shake my sadness all day long. I just wanted to sit
with her at our favorite brewpub, to walk on the old haul road holding
her hand, to sleep with her in the van. The finality of the loss shook

me. I would never be with her again, *ever.* She would never again be here for our wedding anniversary, *ever.* In fact, technically I was no longer even married.

I drank a bottle of wine and retired early, hoping to feel better in the morning. But when I woke up the next day, I felt different, but not better. Instead of sad, I was mad.

I fed the dogs and then drove home to Sacramento. I cancelled dinner with a friend and gave up my $20 ticket to see a good band at the Caspar Inn.

As I left town, I yelled out an obscenity and added, "I am never coming back here again!" I knew I was just venting, but at that moment I really wished we had never bought our land.

After a few days at home, my anger faded. But I wondered how I would feel on subsequent wedding anniversaries.

I talked with Leah a couple of years ago about her spiritual life, and she said she was not worried about her walk with the Lord because he promised he would abide with her no matter what the circumstances. I am sure she and her mom are among the singers who are singing with choirs and praising the Lord.

(Leah's father, Morry)

The final Leah scattering took place the following March. I traveled to Iowa to attend the first Leah Vande Berg Alumni Lecture in Media Studies at the University of Iowa and to visit Leah's family and scatter her ashes on her mother's grave in Sioux Center.

I wanted the lecture to be during Homecoming Week in the fall, but it worked better for the department to schedule it in the spring. By the date of the lecture, it had been 1 year and 4 months since Leah's death. But she was very much on my mind as I boarded the plane.

I did not declare Leah's ashes for fear that officials would not allow me to carry them on the plane. I normally carried her ashes in a brass container, but I knew that container would show up on x-rays. So I put her ashes in a large Vitamin C plastic container, protected it in a Ziploc bag, and stuffed it inside one of my shoes in my suitcase. Not exactly the most dignified way to carry human remains, but at least they made it to Iowa without incident. I also brought a small wooden container to put her ashes in once I arrived.

I flew to Omaha, Nebraska, and felt lucky when the weather was gloomy, but without snow or freezing rain.

I rented a car and headed to Orange City, Iowa, a small town in northwest Iowa where Leah's dad still lived with Leah's stepmother, Hilly. The town is just 8 miles from Sioux Center, Iowa, where Leah was born and raised.

The moment I saw the "Welcome to Iowa" sign I cried, knowing Iowa was the center of Leah's universe and that this was the trip to honor her last request to be scattered on her mother's grave.

Morry and Hilly welcomed me and we visited for a while. Hilly was impressed that I had much shorter hair and real shoes—a pair of Rockports, instead of my usual black tennies. She expressed surprise that I looked good, a surprise that others had expressed throughout the year. I suppose people assumed that I should look as bad as they believed I should feel.

That night I did not sleep well. It was strange staying at Leah's father's house without Leah. I felt as I did the year before—like a walking symbol of Leah's absence, like half of a picture. I had not felt that way in several months.

The next morning, Hilly said Morry did not sleep well either. I'm sure I reminded him of the loss of his daughter.

It was Sunday, so we went to church. Morry introduced me as his son-in-law, which was very nice. Many of their friends expressed condolences. A few older people said they had experienced the loss of their spouses in the last year. One woman added, "So I feel your pain."

We returned to the house, and Hilly's kids and grandchildren came over to celebrate Morry's 79th birthday. Leah's brother, sister-in-law, and niece, Anna Leah, also came. Leah's nephew, Austin, was on a ski trip in Montana.

After lunch and birthday cake, we all headed for the cemetery in Sioux Center. I rode with some of Hilly's kids and answered their questions about Leah's death.

We arrived and waited for everyone to get there. We gathered closely, and I said, "Dear good and gracious God, thank you for Leah, thank you for family and friends."

Morry and Leah's brother, Kevin, also said a few words, although Kevin couldn't finish the passage he was reading and one of Hilly's son-in-laws did so for him.

I told the group that one of Leah's last wishes was for her ashes to be scattered on her mother's grave, and I thanked everyone for helping to honor her request. I stood near Norma's grave, and one by one people walked by, took some ashes, and sprinkled them on the grave. After everyone was finished, I scattered most of the remainder of the ashes over the grave.

Many people cried, and a few sobbed openly. This ceremony was new for them, the funeral that most of them never had, as only Morry, Hilly, and Kevin attended Leah's service. We all stood quietly for a moment, looking at the grave. I held my heart, feeling more emotion than I had felt in many months. I had finally fulfilled my promise to honor Leah's last wishes.

One by one, people offered sympathy and told me how much they loved Leah and missed her. One of Hilly's sons said he had never been to a scattering before, and he thought it was beautiful.

To me the most gratifying aspect was knowing that Leah's family now has a place to go to remember Leah and her mom.

I gave the little box with the remaining ashes to Anna Leah. I asked her to bring them here when Austin came back from Montana so he could scatter his aunt's ashes, too.

The next day, we left for Iowa City. Morry and Hilly led the way in their Cadillac, and Kevin rode with me in my rental car. We talked a lot during the 4-hour drive across the bleak winter landscape. He admitted that he didn't handle some things well, but he said he was doing much better.

The sun broke out by afternoon, but that didn't add much color to the dead trees and dead ground.

One of Leah's former professors took us out to dinner in Iowa City, along with two of Leah's coauthors who would deliver separate lectures for the event.

The lectures were good academic talks that Leah would have appreciated. Morry and Hilly probably were bored, but they were honored about the tribute to Leah.

I was deeply honored to give the first Vande Berg lecture especially because I gave a talk based on the book I was coauthoring with Leah and a colleague. I also was terrified. Leah was deeply committed to the book, and I was concerned that I wouldn't do justice to Leah. I knew her family would be in the audience too, and I was worried that I would be emotional and choke up. I was deeply relieved when I was finished. I also thought it was ironic because I know Leah would have loved being there.

I went through another form of grieving when the book was finished. While I was working on it, Leah was there every day. I could hear her voice and her throaty laugh. The work somehow kept her alive.

But when the book was done, she became a memory. When I received my copies, I thought, this is it. She's gone. I was dismayed.

(Leah's friend and coauthor, Susan)

The day after the lecture, I walked to campus with the Vitamin C container that had the remainder of Leah's ashes. I went to the bookstore to find a little jewelry box with a Hawkeye mascot or something that would be more appropriate for human remains. I could only find a larger wooden box for envelopes, and I asked a clerk whether they had any smaller boxes.

"What do you need it for?" she asked.

I paused. "For my wife's ashes," I said and smiled.

She looked blankly at me.

"Bet you don't get many of those requests," I said.

"Uh, no," she said and quickly rang up my purchase.

I transferred Leah from the vitamin container to the box and went to the communication department. Leah's former professors were not there, so I called her friend, Lucy, who worked in another department. She met me at the river near the old English building where Leah said she wanted to be scattered. Lucy picked a small tree and scattered Leah at its base.

I returned to the department and found one of Leah's former graduate students Jay. We went to the river and he scattered her at the base of a bigger tree. Later I came back one last time with Leah's former professor, Bruce, who scattered Leah in the river. I emptied the rest of the ashes in the river as well.

Bruce went back to his office, but I stayed at the river and said goodbye to Leah. I really felt this was my final goodbye to her.

"I love you so much, Miss Leah," I said. "I miss you. I'm so sorry this happened to you. I learned so much from you. I will always remember you."

I reflected, again, on how important she was in my life and how much of a profound loss her death was for me. I realized that my life would never be the same. I lost my wife, my lover, my best friend, my colleague, my roommate, my everything.

I stayed there for about a half hour, until it started to rain. I could still see a few of her tiny bone fragments in the river near the bank.

When I drove across the Iowa border and back into Nebraska, I said one last goodbye to Leah and to Iowa. I wondered whether I would ever come back to Iowa again.

"Goodbye Miss Leah," I said. "You're in Iowa now. My work is done."

13

Life Really Does Go On

Miss Leah—She wore stylish big hats long before she used them to cover her bald head. It's hard to remember what I noticed first, the full brim straw hat with a long ribbon or her beautiful blue eyes, when we initially met. Leah made an impression on everyone who came into her midst, pulled in by her irresistible smile and then compelled to linger by her strong, steady voice as she would make her position known or invite her listeners on some intriguing revelation of unexplored territory. Over the years, as she became a colleague and then a friend, I grew to value the many gifts she gave to others that helped us all on our own journeys.

Sharing her final days with us was the most precious gift of all. As was her style, dying was not done in some remote sterile way, but in our presence, unencumbered by formalities. We were there when her body was being racked by pain from the deadly cancer that would overtake her, yet even in those difficult last days, she wore her suffering with dignity, managing weak smiles for those she loved, responding to her favorite music and to the sound of Nick's voice. She selected several meaningful songs and messages to be shared at her memorial service, but the one that lingers with me still is . . . , "there's enough love in this room."

Even now, when her physical presence is only a photo of her on my desk, she is with me in my heart, and there's always enough love in the room.

(Leah and Nick's friend and colleague, Marlene)

I know Nick will be fine after I die. He's a young man with another 30 to 40 more years. I am sorry I will not be here with him. I hope he meets somebody who will love him and take care of him and be kind and is wonderful with animals.

To: Friends of Leah
From: nick@csus.edu
Subject: 2nd Anniversary
Date: 12/13/06
    Dear Friends, Relatives, and Colleagues — Today marks the second anniversary of Leah's death. I ask that you take a moment to remember her, especially her smile and her joyous perspective on life.
    In some ways, this anniversary feels like a first one. One year ago, I was in the middle of a 15-month sabbatical and in Australia for my 50th birthday — my first-ever SUMMER birthday. This year I'm home, in the last week of the semester, in the rain and cold, with Christmas decorations everywhere, just as it was two years ago. Of course in other ways it feels like a 5th anniversary. Time does indeed fly by.
    I enjoyed my sabbatical very much. I also traveled to Spain, Morocco, and London this past June. Workwise, I completed a rough first draft of the book with Leah about her cancer and death and my grief, which I continue to work on. At the national convention in November, I organized a panel related to this project, and several people who shared in the experience told their personal stories. The presentation was very moving, and well attended and well received. I left the conference excited to complete this project in the coming year, and I may ask some of you to share your stories for this project.
    Last year at this time, I thought I would teach one more semester and then retire from full-time teaching and move to Ft. Bragg, where I will build a house on my land.
    But I discovered that I love teaching even more than I knew I would. My current plan is to teach

3 to 5 more years and then retire to Ft. Bragg
and pursue international teaching opportunities,
write, paint, play guitar, and do other creative
endeavors, some of which I have started.

Both Leah funds — the Vande Berg Graduate
Scholarship at CSUS and the Vande Berg Alumni
Lecture in Media Studies at the U of Iowa — are
endowed and hopefully will continue to go on every
year. Both funds continue to accept donations, as
the amounts available for the awards each year are
based on the interest generated from the accounts.
Please keep them in mind when you think about
giving donations. Thank you.

I hope you are doing well and that you have
great holidays!

Take care. Love,

nick

There is no substitute for time during the grief process, and sometimes time passes very slowly. Some days in the months that followed Leah's death were agonizingly long. When Leah was alive I stayed up very late—my philosophy then was go to bed in single digits and wake up in double digits. But after her death I wanted to get to sleep as soon as possible, so a new day would start as soon as possible.

But on other days I felt fine. I enjoyed walking the dogs, I started to play tennis again, took up yoga, and did other activities. In fact, on some days I felt so good that I felt guilty about feeling so good, though friends who had gone through similar losses had told me to expect such guilt.

I also started to date again. There is no formula for when a widowed person should date again. In general, men tend to date more quickly than women after the loss of a spouse, but it obviously depends on the person and the situation.

Before I started to date seriously, I told myself not to fall in love with the first person I dated and not to marry the first person I thought I had fallen in love with. I knew I would be very vulnerable, though in retrospect I may have been too rigid about implementing this philosophy.

I first dated a woman I already knew. She was a professor in the field and taught in the Bay Area, a two-hour drive from my house in

Sacramento. I saw her from time to time at conferences, and we were always friendly. I always thought she was very cute and I wanted to ask her out, even though I knew she was at least ten years younger than me. (I learned later she was fifteen years younger).

In April, four months after Leah had died, I tracked down her email address and sent her a note, asking if she'd like to go to lunch or dinner the next time I was in the Bay Area. She replied that she would like to do so, and we agreed on dinner and music.

I used to be nervous when dating, but on the drive to the Bay Area before my first real date I felt unusually calm. I figured that watching my wife of 20 years die was the worst thing I would ever go through in my life. I don't think my death will be as difficult, unless I am eaten alive slowly by ants or starve to death in the desert while pinned under a boulder. So I thought, what's the worst thing that can happen on a date? An awkward pause? A lack of chemistry? She says she doesn't want to see me again?

We had a great time together and agreed to go out again. That date was fun as well, and we went out a few times over the next couple months.

I liked this woman very much, far more than I thought I would, and that worried me. I wasn't sure whether my feelings were genuine or the result of my vulnerability. But I had convinced myself not to fall in love with the first person I dated, so I told her I was not ready for our relationship to continue to develop.

She was upset that I wanted to stop seeing her when we both liked each other and things were going so well. But I just was not yet ready for a relationship.

By then the summer had arrived, as had my sabbatical. I had my choice of taking 1 semester at full pay or 1 year at half pay. Given the insurance money I received, I could easily afford to take the latter, which resulted in a 15-month sabbatical, including the two summers.

Kimo calculated that my sabbatical would be more than 40 million seconds in duration, and he threatened to put a clock on my computer that counted down each second.

After Leah's death, I firmly believe that everyone should, as the expression goes, live for the moment. But it is impossible to live by the second. Just reading this paragraph took several seconds.

I dated another woman on and off for about a month in the summer. I met this second woman through an online dating service that a friend suggested.

I found online dating to be a very interesting experience. My preference was to exchange a few e-mails and then meet at a public place, like a coffee shop, fairly soon to see whether there is any chemistry. Some women who arrived clearly had posted photos from years earlier. I also started to wonder what descriptors like *athletic* really meant.

I did meet one woman a few years older than me, and we had a few good dates. But she was looking for her "soul mate" after a divorce many years earlier, whereas I was just starting to date, so we mutually agreed to stop seeing each other.

Then I dated a woman who taught part time in my department and was working on her master's degree. She was an attractive professional woman in her mid-40s, not the typical 20-something graduate student I dated at Purdue during my brief year of bachelorhood following my divorce. We saw each other at a department party and enjoyed a very fun conversation. On e-mail, I invited her and a few other colleagues and grad students to a concert in the park in July, 7 months after Leah had died.

She was the only person who came to the park, and after the concert we went to dinner. I learned that her father died the day before Leah died, and so we talked openly about our respective losses. We also laughed a lot. We had a fantastic time and agreed to go out again.

We dated a few times in late July and August and quickly fell for each other. In mid-August, I stayed with her for a few days in a rustic cabin at a camp near Yosemite where her family went to fish and ride horses every year. On the first night, we had a drink in an old bar, served by a crusty bartender. Two inebriated deer hunters sat next to us, but fortunately one was a quiet drunk and the other a happy drunk. It was bow-and-arrow season, and they had tracked a deer in the wilderness for a week or so. They finally secured the buck, came back to civilization, and headed straight to the bar. They had been there all day.

The happy drunk saw my date and I flirt with each other, and he told us he was "Doctor Phil" and could help us. He was not the real Doctor Phil, but we thought his attempt to play the role might be amusing.

We engaged in conversation with him for 15 or so minutes, and then I told him we were going to move on.

He looked at me sternly. "No, you don't understand," he said. "I really am Doctor Phil. Tell me the worst thing that ever happened to you and I'll make you feel better."

I looked at my date and said, "Should I?"

She smiled and nodded yes.

"Okay, Doctor Phil," I said, looking into his blood-shot eyes. "Eight months ago my wife died a brutal death from ovarian cancer.

I watched her wither away, and she died before my eyes. Help me out Doctor Phil."

Doctor Phil took a deep breath and tried to regain some sobriety. He took a few seconds and then put his hand on my shoulder.

"I know how you feel," he said tenderly. "My dog died a couple months ago. But she was my hunting dog, so we were real close."

I looked over at my date and smiled. "That is going in the book," I said and laughed.

I thanked Doctor Phil for his counseling session, but I should have thanked him for giving me one of the best examples of what not to say to a widowed person.

The next day, I asked my date to be my girlfriend, and she accepted. And 2 months later, I asked her to join me for a couple weeks during my 4-week trip to Australia. For several years, I had planned to go to Australia for my 50th birthday, although I didn't expect to be there for the first anniversary of my wife's death.

My girlfriend arrived on the first anniversary of her father's death and was with me on the anniversary of Leah's death. I cried very briefly that morning, but being so far away from Sacramento and being with my girlfriend made the anniversary far less painful than I thought it would be.

We had a wonderfully romantic holiday. It felt like a honeymoon, and I nearly asked her to marry me, although I knew I was not ready for that.

We continued to see each other through the spring after a brief breakup, and in June we traveled to Spain, Morocco, and London. But as my wedding anniversary approached, I realized I still had not worked through my feelings of loss related to that date.

I went to Fort Bragg by myself for my wedding anniversary. I was so miserable the year before that I felt I needed to go there to confront my feelings directly so that every July 20 would not be painful.

Although I was a bit sad on the morning of the 20th, I was not depressed or angry, and I did not come home early. But I also felt that July 20 was still my wedding anniversary, and I was not ready to get married again and add another anniversary, although I believe my girlfriend and I were on a track to do just that.

When I returned to Sacramento, I told her about my experience on the north coast and about my feelings. I told her that I could not continue in a relationship that was heading toward marriage. I may have made a mistake, but I simply was not ready for that kind of relationship at that point in time. I probably didn't handle it as well as I could have, but I did what I thought was best for me and for her.

I have dated other women since then, but have not had a serious relationship. As I write these words, Leah has been dead for over 3 years, and only now do I finally feel comfortable being a single man.

I very much would like to get married again, or at least be in a long-term committed relationship. I have had fun dating, but I know I am at my best when I am with a partner. I believe that I will meet the right person some day.

Nick visited us once with a woman he had just started dating. Anything new can be uncomfortable, and we were a little uncomfortable at first. Who is this person? But she was cute and willing to go out with Nick, so we kept our judgments out of it and waited to see how well he liked her. We definitely want him to have his fun. He ended up not seeing her for very long.

I was really happy to see Nick start playing guitar and singing. People often say I wish I would have taken up music earlier, and I always say it's never too late. I think it's good for people to try something new. It's good for healing and for growth. And Nick is totally into it, and his progress has been really good. He digs it and he's having fun.

(Nick's cousin, Pat)

During my sabbatical, I was convinced I would complete my mandatory postsabbatical semester at Sac State and retire from full-time teaching, build my beach house, and live in Fort Bragg for the rest of my life.

But I also knew that a widowed person should not make any rash decisions, so I didn't process any retirement papers. I'm glad I didn't because a funny thing happened on my way to early retirement. I rediscovered that I love my job, my friends, and my life in Sacramento. I still will build my dream house on the north coast, but I have decided to teach full time for a few more years and then make a decision. I believe I will still enjoy a relatively early retirement.

I have made other changes in my life, however. I now am wearing my Rasputin tee shirt again. I almost framed the shirt I wore at the hospital the last weekend, but I decided that would be a somber and somewhat creepy reminder of Leah's death. I decided to wear the shirt again almost 2 years after her death at a panel about the experience at a national communication convention. Jillian was a participant on the panel and had told me that she was going to mention the shirt, so I thought I should wear it. I found it rather amusing that a few people hugged me after the panel and said they were proud of me for wearing that shirt again. It is, after all, just a tee shirt.

More important, I now take at least one international trip every year, something Leah and I never did. Last summer I spent 5 weeks in France, and I hope to go to the Far East and South America in the next few years.

I also started playing guitar and singing. I was always too shy to sing in public, but after watching my wife die I realize the worst thing that can happen is that I am flat or play a wrong chord. I now lead sing-alongs at parties and I'm having a blast. I even have an alter ego named "Gory Bateson," the lead singer of the mythical band "The Ethnogs," whose music videos can be found on YouTube.com.

I also make an effort to help others whose spouses have died. I do not consider myself to be a guardian angel, and I don't read obituaries looking for widows and widowers to call. But when I hear about a friend or acquaintance that suffers the death of a spouse, I contact them. Everyone experiences such a loss in a unique way, but I let them know they are not alone, and I offer to meet with them and tell them about my experience if they wish.

Five people I know have suffered the loss of a spouse since Leah died, and I think I helped each of them at least in some small way. In one case, I have built a friendship that is closer than family.

Lauren was an M.B.A. student who took a graduate class in communication from me more than 15 years ago. She and her husband, Gregory, owned an art gallery and a restaurant, and Leah and I would visit them a few times each year during the "Second Saturday" gallery openings.

Lauren was very kind to me after Leah died, and I would occasionally bring a date to dinner at their restaurant.

Then, in the summer of 2006, I read an obituary about Gregory, who died of esophageal cancer in May of that year. I contributed to the scholarship fund in his honor established by the Art Department at Sacramento State, and I sent Lauren a note saying I would be glad to talk to her if she ever wanted.

She e-mailed me, and we went to lunch a couple months after his death. I also asked whether she would like to read an early excerpt from the book, which she did.

In the years since her husband's death, Lauren and I have become very close friends. I think of her as the older sister I never had, and her restaurant has become my "Cheers Bar," the place where everyone knows my name. I now feel compelled to bring dates there to get my "family's" approval.

Lauren has helped me as much as I have helped her. I had been in Australia for the first anniversary of Leah's death, so as the second one approached it felt more like a first one. I was not feeling good about the anniversary, and I did not want to celebrate my birthday the following day.

Lauren had told me that the anniversary of Leah's death was her wedding anniversary. Because it would be the first wedding anniversary since Gregory's death, I told Lauren I would stop by her restaurant after class to drown our sorrows.

I walked into the restaurant around 8:30 that night, but did not see Lauren at her usual post. A woman sitting at a table with a loud party of eight people asked if I was Nick. I said yes and she shouted out, "He's here."

Lauren brought out a birthday cake and the whole restaurant sang "Happy Birthday" to me. I was a little embarrassed, but mostly touched that Lauren thought of a way to cheer me up, even as she was dealing with her loss on her wedding anniversary.

I went home feeling happy, and I had a great birthday the following day.

The first time I saw Nick after Leah's death, the raw pain in his eyes took my breath away. I could really see how much he was hurting. When I received his card after my husband Gregory's death over a year later, I remembered those eyes. I think that's one reason why I called him. I knew that he really understood what I was feeling because he had gone through a similar experience.

I asked to read an excerpt from his book, and it helped me. I had wondered if things would have been different for Gregory if we had made different decisions about chemotherapy and other aspects of his care. Reading what Nick went through made me realize that these things just happen. It was very comforting.

I have enjoyed watching Nick and his approach to dating. He has been very respectful in discovering what is out there and how he fits into it. He has brought some dates into the restaurant, and although we don't put up flash cards rating the woman as we have joked, we have become a bit protective. It is nice to actually meet and talk to the person and see if they are worthy of him.

It is noteworthy that the anniversary of Leah's death is the same date as our wedding anniversary. Gregory and I never really put much store in anniversary dates. We even had some anniversaries that we entirely forgot about. But the first anniversary after his death felt different I think because people asked me about it and thought it should be different. In a grief situation, dates do serve as reminders. I knew Nick was not feeling very good about the second anniversary of Leah's death and about his birthday, so I wanted to mark the date in a way that was consistent to Nick's approach to getting on. We were respectful of Leah's death and also recognized that his birthday was an important date for him to celebrate.

(Nick's friend, Lauren)

As strange as it may sound—and it still sounds very strange to me—Leah's death was the worst *and* the best thing that ever happened to me. Words will never adequately reveal how brutally horrible it was to watch my wife's body deteriorate and to witness her last breath. But the way she died was truly inspiring, and it definitely changed me. I am not a different person, but I am stronger, kinder, and more joyful.

When Leah was diagnosed with cancer, I wasn't sure whether I could handle what I would go through. In our culture, we are not taught how to care for a dying person or how to grieve. In many ways, we are taught to avoid talking about and dealing with death. But when your spouse—or your parents, friends, or children—are afflicted with a terminal disease, you somehow find a way to deal with it. I now believe that I can handle *anything*, including my own death.

I am also kinder. When you watch your wife die before your eyes, other stuff becomes far less important. I used to take office politics way too seriously, but I have no interest in writing a pissy memo ever again.

I am also more joyous. I really do live my life now according to the credo "Life is Short." I do not take anything for granted. I spend more time doing things I really enjoy. I am more outgoing and sociable, and my circle of friends has expanded. I smile a lot more than I used to, and I have discovered that most people smile back at me.

The only aspect of my life that has not changed for the better since Leah's death is my spiritual life. Although it would be an exaggeration to say that I "lost" faith in God during her cancer and death—as I have considered myself to be a mostly fallen Catholic for many years—my faith in God was weakened, not strengthened, during the experience. I am pleased that Leah's faith in God helped her cope with her illness and death, but I never felt any comfort from Leah's Christian friends and relatives who told me that her death was "part of God's plan." Indeed, I found the idea that God actually decided Leah would die a gruesome death from a horrible disease to be absurd, even morose.

Although I attended services every Sunday with Leah during her illness, I have resumed my old habit of going to church on Christmas and Easter. Organized religion simply has not helped me understand the greater meaning of Leah's death or of my own life and death, nor has it motivated me to search for greater meaning. My perspective before and since Leah's death is that it ultimately comes down to personal faith anyway, regardless of how much you go to church. I do believe there is some kind of next phase after this life, and I believe that what we do in this life does matter, although I don't know what that next phase might be or how what we do in this life might affect that next phase.

I do not know what is in store for me for the rest of my life or after my death. But I will continue to live my life with joy. And I will always remember Miss Leah.

LaVergne, TN USA
03 January 2011
210748LV00005B/20/P